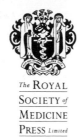

The ROYAL
SOCIETY *of*
MEDICINE
PRESS *Limited*

The Menopause

in Practice

Catrina Bain
Research Fellow, Department of Obstetrics and
Gynaecology, University of Glasgow, UK

Mary Ann Lumsden
Reader in Obstetrics and Gynaecology,
Department of Obstetrics and Gynaecology,
University of Glasgow, UK

Naveed Sattar
Reader in Endocrinology and Metabolism,
Department of Pathological Biochemistry,
University of Glasgow, UK

Ian A Greer
Regius Professor and Head of Department,
Department of Obstetrics and Gynaecology,
University of Glasgow, UK

1 Wimpole Street, London W1G 0AE, UK
207 E Westminster Road, Lake Forest, IL 60045, USA
http://www.rsm.ac.uk

British Library Cataloguing in Publication Data
A catalogue record for this book is available from the British Library

ISBN 1-85315-516-0
ISSN 1473-6845

Phototypeset by Phoenix Photosetting, Chatham, Kent
Printed in Great Britain by Latimer Trend & Company Ltd, Plymouth

About the authors

Catrina Bain MBChB MRCOG is a Specialist Registrar in Obstetrics and Gynaecology in the west of Scotland. She is currently involved in research of the vascular effects of hormone replacement therapy (HRT).

Mary Ann Lumsden MD FRCOG is a Reader in Obstetrics and Gynaecology at the University of Glasgow. She is involved with running the specialist menopause service in Glasgow and has a regular clinical commitment. She is actively involved in clinical research and is particularly interested in the effects of sex steroids on vascular function. She also participates in clinical trials.

Naveed Sattar MBChB PhD MRCPath is a Reader in Endocrinology and Metabolism and Consultant Clinical Biochemist at Glasgow Royal Infirmary University NHS Trust. He has been involved in research in the reproductive arena for 8 years and has published widely on the metabolic changes in relation to pregnancy complications, polycystic ovarian syndrome and HRT. He also conducts research in vascular disease, and has focused recently on the role of inflammatory factors in atherogenesis, including work in major trials such as WOSCOPS and PROSPER.

Ian A Greer MD FRCP(Glas) FRCP(Edin) FRCP (Lond) FRCOG MFFP is Regius Professor and Head of Department of Obstetrics and Gynaecology, University of Glasgow and Honorary Consultant Obstetrician and Gynaecologist, Glasgow Royal Infirmary and Princess Royal Maternity Hospital. His clinical practice focuses on the management of high-risk pregnancies and medical disorders in pregnancy and his research interests focus on vascular function in women and thrombotic problems in obstetrics and gynaecology.

Preface

Management of the menopause is a rapidly changing area. There have been significant developments, particularly with regard to the role of hormone replacement therapy (HRT) and the prevention of coronary heart disease and the risk of venous thromboembolism associated with HRT use. Furthermore, there are alternative strategies for the prevention and treatment of osteoporosis. There is also a diversity of possible therapeutic options for delivering HRT.

The wide range of clinical areas touched on by the menopause and HRT that must be considered in the woman starting or continuing HRT make it difficult for practitioners to keep fully abreast of all the advances in these areas and the implications for management of the menopause. This book aims to provide a succinct review of the current issues relating to the management of the menopause and considers the relevant background science and biology. It steers the reader through advances in areas such as cardiovascular disease, venous thromboembolism, osteoporosis and the various strategies for delivering optimal HRT in a variety of clinical scenarios, and highlights key points and facts. We hope that general practitioners, general gynaecologists and gynaecologists in training will find this volume of value and, perhaps most of all, those that read it enjoy it.

Catrina Bain
Mary Ann Lumsden
Naveed Sattar
Ian A Greer
Glasgow 2002

Contents

1   The menopause: setting the scene   1
Historical perspective   1
Definitions   2
Physiology   3

2   Menopausal symptoms and their management   9
Vasomotor symptoms and sleep disturbance   10
Headache   12
Vaginal atrophy and urinary effects   12
Anxiety and depression   13
Loss of concentration/poor memory   14
Loss of libido   14

3   Premature ovarian failure   17
Diagnosis   17
Psychological effects   18
Osteoporosis   18
Cardiovascular disease   18
Fertility   19
Hormone replacement therapy   19

4   Hormone replacement therapy: preparations and routes of administration   21
The menopause consultation   21
Preparations   23
Oestrogens   24
Progestogens   27
Selective oestrogen receptor modulators   27
Alternative remedies   27

5   Hormone replacement therapy: uptake and suitability   29
Uptake   29
Compliance   30

Side-effects   31
Contraindications   32

6   Osteoporosis   37
Pathogenesis   37
Risk factors   38
Diagnosis   39
Screening and prevention   40
Treatment   42

7   Hormone replacement therapy and arterial disease   49
Protective effect of HRT use   49
Increase in cardiovascular risk with HRT use in prospective randomized trials   49
HRT and blood pressure   52
Current recommendations   52
Prescribing for women at high risk of coronary heart disease   53

8   Hormone replacement therapy and venous thromboembolism   55
HRT-associated risk of venous thromboembolism   55
Relative risk of HRT   57
Recommendations for management   57

9   Hormone replacement therapy and cancer risk   61
Endometrial cancer   61
Breast cancer   63
Ovarian cancer   65
Malignant melanoma   65

Index   67

1. The menopause: setting the scene

Historical perspective
Definitions
Physiology

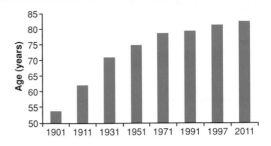

Figure 1.1
Life expectancy in women in the UK, 1901–2011.

The menopause is a complex transition involving biological, psychological, social and cultural factors. Despite advances in understanding of the physiology of menopause, attitudes to the menopause and the management of its symptoms remain polarized. The medical model tends to view the menopause and its associated symptoms as an oestrogen-deficiency state which may require treatment with replacement hormones. The sociocultural perspective views the menopause as a natural part of the life cycle, with menopausal problems being largely socially determined.

Historical perspective

Changes in our lifestyle have greatly influenced our attitude to the cessation of ovarian function and its subsequent effects on women. One of the most important is adjustments in our greater life expectancy. A woman today, with a life expectancy of over 80 years, can expect to spend one-third of her life in the menopausal state.

In evolutionary terms, the menopause is a new phenomenon. Most animals die having reproduced and before ovarian failure. This was also true of humans until improvements in public health increased life expectancy. At the beginning of the 20th century, a woman's average life expectancy at birth was less than 55 years and the proportion of women who survive beyond menopause has significantly increased (Figures 1.1 and 1.2).

> A woman today can expect to spend one-third of her life in the menopausal state

The term 'menopause' is thought to come from the Greek for month (*menos*) and stop (*pausus*).

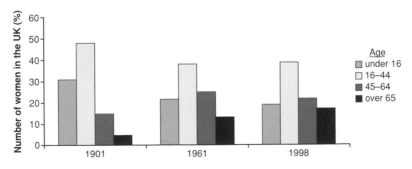

Figure 1.2
Changes in the female population of the UK over the 20th century. (Data source: Social Trends Pocketbook 2000. Office for National Statistics.)

Aristotle noted that menstruation ceased at 40 years. The first reference to the menopause was made by the French physician Gardanne in 1821. It was during the 19th century that the climacteric was increasingly being recognized as a defined event for women, distinct from the gradual decline that occurred in men.

'The transition period, from active ovario-uterine life to the age of sexual decrepitude or degeneration, is seldom effected without some disturbance. Physicians do, indeed, talk of the climacteric in man, but the analogy is more fanciful than real. There is nothing to compare with the sudden decay of the organs of reproduction which marks the middle age of woman.' (Barnes 1873)

'A man grows old by merciful and gentle gradations, and so he slides, half willingly, and half unconsciously, into the afternoon of life ...But for a woman, man's 20 years is compressed into two.' (Charles Reed, President of the American Medical Association 1904)

Victorian attitudes towards menstruation meant that the menopause offered the potential for new freedom: menstruating women were considered to be limited in their ability to function, requiring bed-rest or, at least, refraining from normal activities. In keeping with the attitude that the ovaries were responsible for a woman's psychological weakness, the menopause could be perceived as a positive event if the woman successfully managed to negotiate what was considered to be a precarious phase of life. The Victorian belief that self-restraint in all aspects of life improved health and prevented physical decay, gave a moral perspective to the menopause. Women who experienced significant menopausal symptoms were considered to be suffering as a result of their previous excesses. Menopausal women were advised to *'avoid all such circumstances as might tend to awaken any erotic thought in the mind and reanimate a sentiment that ought rather to become extinct'* (Colombat de L'Isere M. *Treatise on the diseases of females*, 1845).

The remedies recommended for relief of menopausal symptoms have been many and varied, including:

- blood letting
- purgatives
- asses' milk
- raw eggs.

The first idea of hormone replacement therapy (HRT) was proposed in 1888 when Brown-Séquard reported to the Société de Biologie of Paris that he had rejuvenated himself with injections of testicular juice. The use of crude organ extracts, known as organotherapy, became a popular treatment for a wide range of disorders; ovarian therapy for menopausal and other gynaecological symptoms had variable success.

In the early 20th century, the development of fat solvents allowed the isolation of ovarian hormones. By the 1930s, pharmaceutical companies had developed natural and synthetic hormones that gradually superseded organotherapy. The efficacy of HRT as a treatment for the menopause did not become established within mainstream medical opinion until the 1960s. Since then, its use has increased, apart from a period in the 1980s when it became apparent that unopposed oestrogen use was associated with endometrial carcinoma. The subsequent addition of progesterone improved safety and the uptake of HRT has slowly increased since the 1980s but remains low in the UK.

Definitions

The menopause

The menopause is defined retrospectively as the occurrence of the last menstrual period. The World Health Organization describes the menopause as the permanent cessation of menstruation resulting from the loss of ovarian follicular activity. The period of 'transition', which heralds the decline of ovarian function, can often cause problematical symptoms even though menstruation continues. Many women commence HRT around this time for amelioration of symptoms, which often causes confusion over the date of the last menstrual period due to withdrawal bleeding.

The menopause transition or perimenopause

The menopausal transition or perimenopause is less clearly defined but is generally regarded as being characterized by menstrual irregularity associated with other menopausal symptoms. This phase is completed when menstruation ceases. Only about 10% of women cease menstruation rapidly; for most the menopausal transition lasts around 4 years.

> The menopausal transition or perimenopause lasts around 4 years

Age at menopause

Studies of the age at menopause have often relied on patient recall, with obvious limitations.

The average age at which the menopause occurs in western Caucasian populations is 51–52 years. Studies of menopause in different populations suggest that it occurs earlier for non-Caucasian women. The method of data collection varies between studies and may contribute to perceived differences in age of menopause. A community-based survey of 14,620 women within seven North American centres suggested that race has an influence on menopausal age: African and Hispanic women had a slightly earlier natural menopause and Japanese women slightly later when compared with Caucasian women.

Some studies have suggested that socioeconomic factors may moderately reduce the age at menopause, including:

- low educational status
- not being married
- not being employed.

A consistent finding is that smoking reduces the age of menopause by 1–2 years (Figure 1.3). Use of oral contraceptives and increased parity may be associated with a later menopause. The timing of the natural menopause tends to be inherited, with daughters experiencing the menopause around the same time as their mothers.

> The menopause occurs at an average age of 51–52 years in western Caucasian women

Premature menopause

A premature menopause occurs in 1% of women and is defined as the menopause before the age of 45 years (see Chapter 3). In many ways, this is a different entity from a natural menopause, with additional factors to be considered, such as infertility and the psychological consequences of what may be perceived as premature ageing.

Genetic defects can be responsible for premature menopause and a range of conditions, including iatrogenic causes, can influence ovarian ageing. Women who experience a premature menopause have higher risks of cardiovascular disease and osteoporosis.

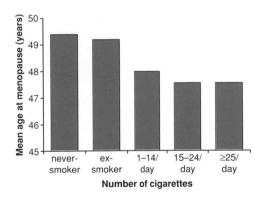

Figure 1.3
Number of cigarettes smoked and mean age at menopause.

1% of women experience a premature menopause

The average age of menopause is younger in women who have undergone a hysterectomy

Surgical menopause

A surgical menopause is defined as surgical cessation of menses by removal of the uterus and both ovaries. Postoperatively these women have a very rapid decline in circulating hormone levels and are more likely to experience severe symptoms when compared to women who have undergone a natural menopause. A woman who has her ovaries conserved during hysterectomy can usually expect them to function as normal; however, menopause can occur prematurely, possibly because the blood supply to the ovary is affected by the operation. This results in an overall earlier age at menopause for women who have undergone hysterectomy.

The lack of menses can make diagnosis of the menopause more difficult and this is an occasion where measurement of gonadotrophin levels may be helpful.

Physiology

The normal function of the ovary is to produce steroid hormones and to release the oocyte in response to stimulation from the gonadotrophins, luteinizing hormone (LH) and follicle-stimulating hormone (FSH).

A finite number of oocytes are produced during intrauterine life and, unlike spermatogenesis, no further development occurs. The follicle passes through a number of distinct developmental phases prior to ovulation (Figure 1.4). The most immature stage is termed 'primordial' – a small oocyte surrounded by a single layer of granulosa cells. The oocyte is arrested during the first meiotic division and no further development takes place until many years later, just prior to ovulation.

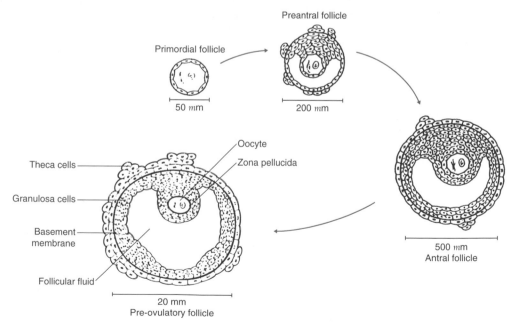

Figure 1.4
Developing follicle.

During the normal menstrual cycle, several of the primordial follicles will be recruited and will develop in preparation for ovulation. There is a dramatic increase in size as well as proliferation of the surrounding granulosa cells. Production of sex steroids increases and a large fluid-filled antrum develops. Antral development requires stimulation by gonadotrophins and, prior to puberty, the FSH levels are insufficient to sustain follicular development beyond the primordial state.

Only the dominant follicle continues to develop. This process and the selection of a follicle is poorly understood. Only around 400 follicles will actually mature and ovulate during an average woman's reproductive lifetime, with the vast majority defaulting to atresia.

There are between one and two million oocytes present within the ovary at birth. The number of follicles within the ovary declines with age with a steady, gradual decline between birth and the age of 37 years and a rapid decline beyond 37 years (Figure 1.5). It has been estimated that, if the initial slow rate of decline continued, the menopause would occur at the age of 70. The rate of decline does not appear to be affected by processes that halt ovulation, such as pregnancy, lactation or the contraceptive pill.

Luteinizing hormone and FSH are produced by the anterior pituitary in response to pulsatile production of gonadotrophin-releasing hormone by the hypothalamus. The production of oestradiol by the ovary has a largely negative feedback effect on the pituitary and hypothalamus. The low level of oestrogen that is present during menstruation results in a rise in the FSH levels. This causes development of the follicle and the production of oestrogen, initiating development of the endometrium with growth of arterioles and glandular tissue. By the end of the follicular phase, the rising oestradiol levels have a positive feedback effect, producing the LH surge which causes ovulation. The corpus luteum then produces progesterone and during the secretory phase the arterioles develop further and glandular tissue increases,

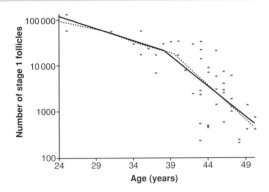

Figure 1.5
Number of oocytes present during a woman's life.

becoming tortuous and oedematous. These changes (Figure 1.6) prepare the endometrium for implantation of the developing zygote. If pregnancy fails to occur, the corpus luteum degenerates within 10–14 days, production of oestrogen and progesterone declines and menstruation occurs a few days later.

Menstruation

The exact mechanisms for menstruation are complex but it appears that the withdrawal of oestrogen and progesterone is crucial to the process. The fall in hormone levels is associated with constriction of the spiral arterioles and the endometrium is subsequently shed.

In the first few years after the menarche, ovulation has not become established and the bleeding pattern is characterized by long cycles. This is because of prolonged stimulation by oestrogen with no progestogenic effect to induce a regular bleed. The endometrium then breaks down in an irregular fashion and the resulting bleed can be prolonged and heavy. Once ovulation has become established and regular menstrual cycles occur, this usually continues until a women reaches her early 40s.

Age-related changes in menstrual cycle

The initial change in the menstrual cycle, which occurs as women age, tends to be a slightly

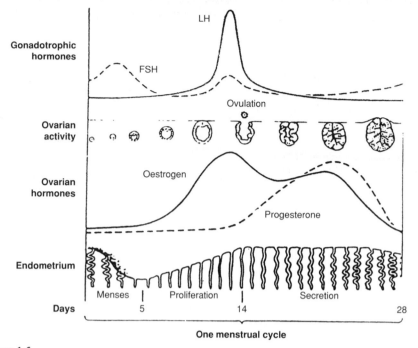

Figure 1.6
Changes in FSH, LH, oestrogen, progesterone and the endometrium during the normal menstrual cycle.

shorter cycle length. This pattern tends to occur in the late 30s and early 40s. The secretory phase of the cycle remains constant with the follicular phase becoming shorter. There is a trend towards an increase in FSH levels in the follicular phase of the cycle. This occurs even when oestradiol levels are unchanged and ovulation continues. A study of 500 infertile women with regular cycles noted that this increase in follicular FSH occurred around the age of 37 years, although it may take place as early as 29–30 years.

> The length of the menstrual cycle shortens slightly in women in their late 30s/early 40s

The developing follicle produces a glycoprotein hormone inhibin (subtypes A and B) which appears to inhibit FSH selectively and may be involved in the regulation of ovulation. Inhibin A levels are highest in the luteal phase of the cycle, and inhibin B levels are highest in the

follicular phase and around ovulation. As women age, the level of circulating inhibins gradually falls, reflecting the rate of ovarian ageing.

The menopause transition and the menopause

Menstrual pattern

The menopause transition is characterized by irregular menstrual cycles in association with menopausal symptoms. As the menopause approaches, the hormone levels are more likely to fluctuate leading to irregular bleeding. With ovarian ageing, the ability to develop a follicle fully for ovulation declines and menstrual cycles are also more likely to be anovulatory. During these cycles, oestrogen causes continued endometrial development, but there is no progesterone production to induce a regular period. This typically causes prolonged erratic cycles and, when the menstrual bleed does occur, it can be heavier and more prolonged than usual. This pattern can be interspersed with relatively regular, ovulatory episodes.

As the numbers of ovulations are reduced, the chance of successful conception is lower but the actual reasons for reduced fertility in this age group are more complex with oocyte ageing affecting function.

> During the menopausal transition, the menstrual cycle is often longer and erratic, with prolonged and heavier bleeding

The last menstrual period is identified retrospectively. The older a woman is, the more likely it is that a period of amenorrhoea reflects a genuine menopausal state.

Hormone levels

In the premenopausal woman, the two major oestrogens produced are oestradiol and the less biologically potent oestrone. In the postmenopausal woman, the production of oestrogenic hormones falls; however, the ovarian stroma continues to produce androstendione, which is converted peripherally by adipose tissue to low levels of oestradiol and oestrone. Obese postmenopausal women have higher endogenous oestrogen levels than non-obese postmenopausal women.

A prospective study of the hormone profile in perimenopausal women showed that oestradiol levels remained relatively constant until 6 months prior to the last menstrual period. The decline in oestradiol was associated with a significant increase in FSH and a smaller increase in LH levels.

However, the hormone profile is generally an unhelpful investigation in perimenopausal women. Levels of both oestradiol and FSH do not always correlate well with menopausal symptoms and fluctuate significantly from pre- to post-menopausal values on an almost daily

basis in the perimenopause. If a woman has a history of flushes and sweats or associated mood disturbance together with menstrual irregularity, she should be considered to be perimenopausal. Regardless of hormonal status, she is likely to obtain benefit from HRT if menopausal symptoms are a problem.

> The hormone profile is often an unhelpful investigation in perimenopausal women

Once ovarian function ceases completely, amenorrhoea persists and the FSH level remains elevated (>30 IU/l is diagnostic). LH levels rise to a lesser extent and it should be remembered that a high LH level in a perimenopausal woman may reflect an ovulatory LH surge. Ovarian production of oestradiol declines significantly; however, conversion of androstendione by peripheral tissues will produce low levels of estrone that are converted to oestradiol.

The doses of oestrogens in standard HRT are not high enough to suppress ovulation and a woman should be considered potentially fertile for 2 years after her last menstrual period if she is under 50 years of age, and for 1 year if she is over 50 years.

Further reading

Ahmed Ebbiary NA, Lenton EA, Cooke ID. Hypothalamic-pituitary ageing: progressive increase in FSH and LH concentrations throughout reproductive life of regularly menstruating women. Clin Endocrinol 1994; 41: 199–206.

Burger HG, Dudley EC, Hopper JL et al. The endocrinology of the menopausal transition: a cross sectional study of a population based sample. J Clin Endocrinol Metab 1996; 81: 3537–45.

Gold EB, Bromberger J, Crawford S et al. Factors associated with age at natural menopause in a multiethnic sample of midlife women. Am J Epidemiol 2001; 153: 865–74.

Hayes FJ, Hall JE, Boepple PA et al. Differential control of gonadotrophin secretion in the human: endocrine role of inhibin. J Clin Endocrinol Metab 1998; 83: 1835–41.

Kaufan DW, Slone D, Rosenburg L et al. Cigarette smoking and age at natural menopause. Am J Pub Health 1980; 70: 420–1.

McKinlay SM, Brambilla DJ, Posner JG. The normal menopausal transition. *Maturitas* 1992; **14**: 102–15.

Moscucci O. Medicine, age and gender: the menopause in history. *J Br Menopause Soc* 1999; **5**: 149–53.

Rannevik G, Jeppsson S, Johnell O *et al*. A longitudinal study of the peri-menopausal transition: altered profiles of steroid and pituitary, SHBG and bone mineral density. *Maturitas* 1995; **21**: 103–13.

Reidel HH, Lehmann-Willenbrock E, Semm K. Ovarian failure after hysterectomy. *J Reprod Med* 1986; **31(7)**: 597–600.

Richardson SJ, Senikas V, Nelson JF. Follicular depletion during the menopausal transition: evidence for accelerated loss and ultimate exhaustion. *J Clin Endocrinol Metab* 1987; **65**: 1231–7.

Sherman BM, Korenman SG. Hormonal characteristics of the human menstrual cycle throughout reproductive life. *J Clin Invest* 1975; **55**: 699–706.

Siddle N, Sarrel P, Whitehead M. The effect of hysterectomy on the age at ovarian failure: identification of a subgroup of women with premature loss of ovarian function and literature review. *Fertil Steril* 1987; **47(1)**: 94–100.

Torgerson DJ, Thomas RE, Reid DM. Mothers' and daughters' menopausal ages: is there a link? *Eur J Obstet Gynecol Reprod Biol* 1997; **74**: 63–6.

Utian WH. Historical perspectives in menopause. Menopause. *J Am Menopause Soc* 1999; **6(2)**: 83–6.

2. Menopausal symptoms and their management

**Vasomotor symptoms and sleep
   disturbance
Headache
Vaginal atrophy and urinary effects
Anxiety and depression
Loss of concentration/poor memory
Loss of libido**

Symptoms are experienced by approximately 80% of women in the UK during the menopausal transition and include:

- hot flushes
- palpitations
- night sweats
- sleep disturbance
- vaginal dryness
- urinary urgency
- depressed mood
- irritability
- lethargy
- forgetfulness and loss of concentration
- loss of libido.

For some women, these symptoms may be relatively mild and short lasting, but for others, the menopause can cause significant physical and psychological morbidity. This chapter discusses the individual symptoms associated with the menopause and outlines briefly the therapeutic measures that might be taken. Hormone replacement therapy is covered in depth in Chapters 4 and 5.

> 80% of women in the UK experience menopausal symptoms

Socioeconomic factors

In common with other medical conditions, a woman's social circumstances may affect how she perceives and copes with the menopause transition. Typically, the menopause can coincide with a time in a woman's life when she may face significant life events:

- 'empty nest' syndrome with offspring leaving home
- marital difficulties
- development of age-related illnesses
- infirmity of parents.

The social model of the menopause hypothesizes that these changes may be directly responsible for psychological symptoms, such as depressed mood or irritability, that are commonly reported during the climacteric and which alter perception of physical symptoms.

Surveys have shown that women in employment have fewer problems with menopausal symptoms than those not in employment. A community-based survey of Australian women found fewer menopausal symptoms with longer years of education, a lower level of stress, non-smoking, regular exercise, the absence of chronic health conditions and positive attitudes to menopause and ageing.

The relationship between menopausal symptoms and social status is complex. Women who attend specialist clinics for menopausal symptoms are more likely to be suffering from psychosocial stress, although the frequency of hot flushes and vaginal atrophy is similar to that of postmenopausal women who are not attending a menopause clinic. It is likely that some women are more prone to psychological effects of hormone fluctuations than others. There is certainly a relationship between premenstrual disorders and the experience of a more difficult menopause.

Racial and cultural differences

Racial differences are known to impact on the menopausal experience. More research is needed, including studies of different racial groups, as most evidence is based on Caucasian women in developed countries. This is being addressed by ongoing randomized controlled trials, which are recruiting a representative mix of racial backgrounds.

Cultural differences can affect a woman's perceptions of the menopause. In the West, youth and beauty are highly valued and fertility is closely linked to these attributes. In many developing cultures, the menopause relieves a woman of the burden of fertility and can be a time of greater freedom. Menstruation has considerable social limitations in some societies. These limitations are removed at the time of menopause and continued vaginal bleeding from HRT may be even less acceptable than it is to Western women. In Oriental and Asian cultures, menstruating women are perceived as not clean and certain activities are forbidden to them, including religious activities, swimming and sexual intercourse.

In some cultures, older age is associated with greater status in society and the menopause can be welcomed as a positive event. Within Asian communities, older women have greater freedom and status than their younger counterparts, and housework becomes less of a burden as daughters and daughters-in-law take care of the household.

There appears to be some cultural variation in the experience of the menopause. Reporting of menopausal symptoms is very different, with much lower rates of hot flushes being described by Oriental women when compared to Western women. The Mayan Indian population has a very low incidence of menopausal problems and the Mayan language has no word for hot flush. A recent community-based survey of menopausal symptoms in the US compared the menopausal experience for different ethnic groups. This found that:

- women of African origin reported more vasomotor and vaginal dryness
- Hispanic women were more likely to report urogenital symptoms, palpitations and forgetfulness
- Oriental women were less likely to complain of all menopausal symptoms.

It may be that there are genuine differences in the individual experience of such symptoms. One mechanism postulated to be responsible for this is the level of phytoestrogens (plant oestrogens) in the diet. There may be other reasons, as not all studies have shown such low levels and there appear to be differences among different social groups within developing countries, with affluent members of a developing society experiencing more menopausal problems. It is possible that some cultures do not encourage menopausal women to complain of symptoms.

Vasomotor symptoms and sleep disturbance

Hot flushes – the classic menopausal symptom – are experienced by up to 80% of women at some time related to the menopause and are a significant problem for up to 45%. They are characterized by an intermittent sensation of heat, flushing and perspiration, usually affecting the face, neck and chest. Many women report a prodromal phase, often describing a pressure sensation in the head. For some, flushing can be associated with palpitations or feeling faint.

The flushes usually occur spontaneously, although some factors may provide a trigger, eg stressful situations, spicy foods, alcohol or caffeine. The lack of predictability of flushing can be distressing for women who feel a lack of control and often report feelings of embarrassment.

> Hot flushes are a significant problem for up to 45% of women

Demonstrable physiological changes occur prior to the subjective complaint. The first sign is dilatation of vessels within the skin, followed by a rise in skin temperature and an increase in perspiration. Pulse rate increases slightly and core temperature falls; some women report a chilled sensation at the end of the flushing episode.

The exact cause of hot flushes is not clear but the likely mechanism is thought to be the response of the hypothalamus to the low oestrogen levels, resulting in higher levels of neurotransmitters, including noradrenaline. This leads to a resetting of the thermoregulatory centre. Gonadotrophin levels are unimportant – patients on gonadotrophin-releasing analogues have very low levels of circulating gonadotrophins but do experience flushing.

The change in oestrogen levels appears to be more important than the absolute value: prepubertal and many elderly women have low levels of oestrogens but do not experience flushing symptoms; women with primary hypogonadism do not experience flushes unless they have first been exposed to exogenous oestrogen. In common with many other menopausal symptoms, vasomotor symptoms are experienced most by women in the perimenopausal phase when oestrogen levels are fluctuating, and tend to decline the further a woman is from her last menstrual period. Women who undergo a surgical menopause have a precipitous fall in hormone levels and tend to experience more severe hot flushes when compared to women who undergo a natural menopause. Women who experience a tachyphylaxis with high-dose oestradiol implants can have hot flushes even when the oestradiol levels are above premenopausal values.

Hot flushes occurring at night are known as night sweats. Insomnia is a common feature of vasomotor problems at night with women frequently reporting the unpleasant sensation of waking, drenched in sweat, to the extent that bedclothes need to be changed. In the long term, sleep disturbance can contribute to fatigue and psychological effects, particularly loss of concentration and mood swings. Objective assessment of sleep patterns in women with night sweats has shown that waking episodes sometimes occur before the flush and the sleep disturbance may be more complex than simply the discomfort produced by the temperature changes and perspiration. Sleep disturbance can occur without apparent vasomotor symptoms.

> Sleep disturbance can contribute to psychological effects

Management

Oestrogen has clearly been demonstrated by many randomized controlled trials to treat hot flushes effectively and remains the gold standard therapy. Other options include progestogens, which have been shown to reduce flushing, although to a much lesser extent. Clonidine, a centrally active alpha-blocker has also been shown to reduce flushes in short-term trials (8 weeks or less). As with progestogens, clonidine is less effective at treating vasomotor symptoms when compared to oestrogen but both of these options may be considered for women where oestrogen is contraindicated.

Antidepressants can reduce menopausal flushes for some women. A placebo-controlled trial of venlafaxine in women with breast cancer has been shown to reduce menopausal flushes. Dose-related side-effects such as dry mouth, decreased appetite, nausea and constipation were significantly more common in patients on venlafaxine. It was suggested that a starting dose should be 37.5 mg daily, increasing to 75 mg daily if required.

Women frequently report an improvement in their sleep pattern with hormone replacement therapy (HRT) even when flushes or night sweats are not a feature of their menopausal symptoms.

Headache

Headache and, in particular, migraine appears to be associated with fluctuating hormone levels:

- Perimenstrual migraine is well documented.
- Migraine sometimes worsens in the first trimester of pregnancy, but is usually less frequent in the last two trimesters when the hormone levels are at their peak.
- Postnatally, headache frequency, again, increases at a time when hormone levels have fallen.

Headache and exacerbation of migraine is also a frequent perimenopausal complaint. There is no evidence that migraine in a woman aged over 45 years is a risk factor for stroke and there is no contraindication to use of HRT for women with migraine.

> Headache and exacerbation of migraine is a frequent perimenopausal complaint

Management

For women who experience an exacerbation of headache perimenopausally, use of HRT can provide stable hormone levels and improve symptoms. However, HRT can exacerbate migraine in a small proportion of women; this is usually dose-related in women who are particularly sensitive to the effects of hormones. For these women, a reduction in dose of oestrogen or a change in route of delivery can be effective. A transdermal preparation often delivers a lower dose at a steady rate when compared to an oral preparation. Initially, the lowest dose should be used with a gradual increase until the patient's symptoms are controlled.

The progestogen component of HRT can cause headache through the mineralocorticoid effect and its associated fluid-retention effect. An alternative progestogen or a different route of administration with less systemic absorption, such as vaginal progesterone or the levonorgestrel-containing intrauterine system (LNG-IUS), can lead to an improvement in symptoms.

Vaginal atrophy and urinary effects

The female genital and lower urinary tracts share a common embryological origin and are highly sensitive to the effects of oestrogen. Oestrogen receptors are found in many tissues throughout the pelvis, including:

- mucosa
- smooth muscle
- voluntary muscle
- ligaments.

Well-oestrogenized vaginal mucosa is a thick tissue with abundant glycogen-rich cells. It interacts with lactobacilli to produce an acidic vaginal pH, which helps prevent infection.

Oestrogen deprivation results in a thin, dry mucosa. The rugae of the vagina disappear and the vagina shortens after the menopause. There is a reduction in lactic acid formation with a resulting rise in vaginal pH, leading to bacterial overgrowth. The thin mucosa, lack of lubrication and increased susceptibility to infection together cause a range of symptoms, including localized discomfort, a burning or itching sensation, dyspareunia and discharge.

Atrophy of the periurethral tissues can contribute to symptoms of frequency and urgency and predispose to urinary tract infection. The timing of urogenital symptoms in relationship to the menopause varies: some women experience atrophic changes perimenopausally but for the majority, urogenital symptoms occur several years after the menopause.

> Urogenital symptoms tend to occur several years after the menopause

Management

Vaginal dryness can be treated simply with topical oestrogen therapy or systemic HRT. The route of administration will depend on the patient's age and other symptoms. Atrophic changes are frequently detected in older women who attend for other reasons such as assessment of vaginal prolapse or for the change of a ring pessary. A topical oestrogen with minimal systemic absorption is the preferred option in this case.

The mucosa of the urogenital tract responds well to a low dose of oestrogen. Little systemic absorption occurs with these doses, minimizing unwanted systemic side-effects and endometrial hyperplasia. The options for administration include vaginal tablets, creams or ring pessaries. The tablets and creams should be used on an intermittent basis after an initial 2–3 week course of daily application. Low-dose ring pessaries that release as little as 7.5 μg of oestradiol daily are available.

A woman with vaginal atrophy in addition to other symptoms requires systemic HRT. However, the option of vaginal administration is now available and avoids the first-pass metabolism of an oral route (see Chapter 4). Significant quantities of oestradiol can be absorbed through the vaginal mucosa, providing systemic levels to relieve symptoms but, like other systemic oestrogens, endometrial hypertrophy is a risk in a women with a uterus unless progesterone is given. These issues are discussed in greater depth in Chapter 4.

With regard to urinary incontinence, the evidence of objective improvement with HRT is conflicting. Most studies have shown little benefit in stress incontinence, although there may be a case for treating women with mild stress incontinence conservatively with oestrogens. Urge incontinence appears to be more amenable to treatment with HRT. Subjective improvement of urge incontinence has been demonstrated when treated with topical oestrogens.

For women with recurrent urinary tract infection, vaginal oestrogens significantly reduce the rate of infection when compared to placebo.

Anxiety and depression

Mood and anxiety have a complex relationship with female hormones:

- The incidence of depression is approximately twice as high in women as it is in men.
- During the reproductive years, cyclical fluctuations in hormones are associated with premenstrual mood disorder and postnatal depression is associated with the dramatic fall in hormonal levels after delivery. A British community survey has shown higher rates of depression in women throughout the reproductive years than in those over the age of 55 years.
- There is little evidence of higher rates of major depression among postmenopausal women and the levels of circulating hormones are no different in depressed women when compared to those who are not depressed.

Some studies have shown that the perimenopausal phase is associated with a higher rate of depression and it does appear that women are at their most vulnerable when hormone levels are fluctuating.

It is likely that mild mood changes may arise during the menopause, particularly when other symptoms are present. Patients with a history of depression have a higher risk of menopausal mood disorders. However, it is difficult to separate this relationship from that between other menopausal symptoms and depression; sleep deprivation is a common feature of the menopause and this, together with other symptoms, can affect a woman's ability to cope with life events. Menopausal women may also be facing social changes, which can affect mood and sense of wellbeing.

> Patients with a history of depression have a higher risk of menopausal mood disorders

Oestrogen has many positive effects on the brain – it decreases the breakdown of neurotransmitters, such as serotonin, and increases their production – and may have a 'mental tonic' effect that improves mood in a general sense. A study of asymptomatic postmenopausal women demonstrated that oestrogen improved mood when compared to placebo. There is a close relationship between mood disorders in the menopause and the premenstrual syndrome: women who experience mood changes in association with falling hormone levels of the late luteal phase are prone to mood disorder in the menopause.

Management

Relatively high doses of oestrogen have been shown to be effective in treating women with severe depression. One study randomized pre- and post-menopausal women with major depressive disorders to increasing doses of conjugated oestrogens or placebo and found significant improvement in the oestrogen group. These patients were described as severely depressed, therapy-resistant women in whom very low rates of spontaneous remission could be expected.

Although it should not be assumed that a woman is depressed because she is menopausal, there is a case for using HRT in women in the perimenopausal or menopausal phase as a first-line option, assuming there is no contraindication. If other menopausal symptoms are also a feature, the chances of successful treatment are higher with HRT.

Counselling should be considered together with the use of antidepressants when required.

Loss of concentration/poor memory

Frequent complaints among menopausal women are an inability to concentrate and an impaired short-term memory. These are highly subjective problems that may be related to other menopausal symptoms such as flushes or sleep disturbance.

There is some evidence that hormonal status has an impact on cognitive ability:

- Studies of cognition in menopausal women have shown that current and previous users of HRT have higher scores in measures of cognitive ability, particularly verbal learning and memory.
- Randomized controlled trials comparing HRT users with non-users have demonstrated an improvement in cognitive functioning for women who were experiencing menopausal symptoms, but no clear benefit for women without menopausal symptoms.

Possible mechanisms include increased activity of neurotransmitters [particularly serotonin, norepinephrine (noradrenaline) and dopamine], effect on neurite and synaptic reorganization or possibly direct vascular effects.

Management

It is appropriate to consider HRT for improvement of cognitive symptoms, particularly where other menopausal symptoms are present. There are, however, many other factors that affect cognitive ability.

Loss of libido

Loss of libido is a relatively frequent complaint among menopausal women. It is a complex issue: many factors relevant to middle life can affect sexuality, particularly social change and sexual difficulties of male partners. Other menopausal symptoms such as night sweats, mood changes and vaginal dryness may adversely affect sexual function.

Management

Time spent exploring relevant issues can be productive and formal counselling sessions are worth considering as there are many factors that can be involved (see Table 2.1).

The role of standard oestrogen-based HRT for the management of loss of libido is debatable when this is the only menopausal complaint. Some women do respond to oestrogen replacement, but it may be that the relief of other symptoms leads to an improvement in libido rather than there being a direct effect.

For both men and women, androgens have an important role in sexual function. A gradual decrease in levels of circulating androgens begins in the years before the menopause and continues as women age. There is no sudden drop as occurs with oestrogens at the menopause. After the menopause, the ovaries continue to produce androgens and women who have undergone bilateral oophorectomy at hysterectomy have very low circulating androgen levels. Androgen supplementation can improve libido for some women, particularly those who have undergone oophorectomy.

In the UK, testosterone is available for women only as subcutaneous implants. As testosterone can have adverse effects on lipids, it is recommended that both serum lipids and liver function are confirmed as normal before a course of treatment is started. New methods of administration are being developed.

Tibolone, a synthetic steroid, has partial oestrogenic, progestogenic and androgenic properties. It may improve libido for some women and is worth considering for a woman who requires management of vasomotor symptoms and loss of libido.

Table 2.1
Factors to consider and treatment options in the management of loss of libido in the menopause

Factors to consider:
- Social circumstances
- Psychological effects of the menopause
- Male partner: erectile dysfunction
- Other menopausal symptoms
- History of sexual problems

Treatment options:
- Counselling
- Topical oestrogens if vaginal dryness is present
- Systemic HRT if vasomotor, mood swings, etc, are present
- Tibolone
- Testosterone implants

Further reading

Bebbington PE, Dunn G, Jenkins R et al. The influence of age and sex on the prevalence of depressive conditions: a report from the National Survey of Psychiatric Morbidity. Psychol Med 1998; **28**: 9–19.

Dennerstein L, Smith AM, Morse C et al. Menopausal symptoms in Australian women. Med J Aust 1993; **159**: 232–6.

Ditkoff EC, Crary WG, Cristo M et al. Estrogen improves psychological function in asymptomatic postmenopausal women. Obstet Gynecol 1991; **78(6)**: 991–5.

Fantl JA, Cardozo LD, McClish DK and the Hormones and Urogenital Therapy Committee. Oestrogen therapy in the management of incontinence in postmenopausal women: a meta-analysis. First report of the Hormones and Urogenital Therapy Committee. Obstet Gynecol 1994; **83**: 12–18.

Gold EB, Sternfield B, Kelsey JL et al. Relationship of demographic and lifestyle factors to symptoms in a multi-racial/ethnic population of women 40–55 years of age. Am J Epidemiol 2000; **152**: 463–73.

Greendale GA, Lee NP, Arriola ER. The menopause. Lancet 1999; **353**: 571–80.

Klaiber EL, Broverman DM, Vogel W et al. Estrogen therapy for severe persistent depression in women. Arch Gen Psych 1979; **36**: 550–4.

Loprinzi CL, Michalak JC, Quella SK et al. Megestrol acetate for the prevention of hot flushes. N Engl J Med 1994; **331(6)**: 347–52.

Loprinzi CL, Kugler JW, Sloan JA et al. Venlafaxine in the management of hot flashes in survivors of breast cancer: a randomised controlled trial. Lancet 2000; **356**: 2059–63.

Le Blanc ES, Janowsky J, Chan BK et al. Hormone replacement therapy and cognition: systematic review and meta-analysis. JAMA 2001; **285**: 1489–99.

McKinlay JB, McKinlay SM, Brambilla DJ. Health status and utilisation behaviour associated with menopause. Am J Epidemiol 1987; **125**: 110–21.

Porter M, Penney GC, Russell D et al. A population based survey of women's experience of the menopause. Br J Obstet Gynaecol 1996; **103**: 1025–8.

Raz R, Stamm WE. A controlled trial of intravaginal estriol in postmenopausal women with recurrent urinary tract infections. N Engl J Med 1993; **329**: 736–60.

Rymer J, Morris P. Menopausal symptoms. Br Med J 2000; **321**: 1516–19.

Silberstein S, Merriam G. Sex hormones and headache 1999 (menstrual migraine). Neurology 1999; **53**: 3–13.

Soares CN, Almeida OP, Joffe H et al. Efficacy of oestradiol for treatment of depressive disorders in perimenopausal women: a double-blind, randomised, placebo-controlled trial. Arch Gen Psychiat 2001; **58(6)**: 537–8

3. Premature ovarian failure

Diagnosis
Psychological effects
Osteoporosis
Cardiovascular disease
Fertility
Hormone replacement therapy

Premature ovarian failure (POF) is rare among young women but rises to 1% of western women by the age of 40 years. It is an heterogeneous condition with most cases thought to be idiopathic. Several factors can, however, result in premature interruption of ovarian function (Table 3.1).

> Most cases of premature ovarian failure are idiopathic

POF can be classified as due to either premature depletion of follicles or to follicle dysfunction, in which normal oocytes and follicles appear to be present but they are resistant to adequate levels of gonadotrophins. The latter condition is also referred to as 'resistant ovary syndrome'. Ovarian biopsy has not been found to be helpful in the diagnosis or prediction of remission.

> Premature ovarian failure is due either to premature depletion of follicles or to follicle dysfunction

Diagnosis

Women usually present with amenorrhoea and the diagnosis of a premature menopause is based upon an elevated follicle-stimulating hormone (FSH) level (>30 mIU/ml) together

Table 3.1
Causes of premature ovarian failure (POF)

Genetic	Turner's syndrome
	X chromosome abnormalities
	Down's syndrome
	Mutation of the follicle-stimulating hormone (FSH) receptor
	Specific enzyme deficiencies
	Galactosaemia
Surgical	Bilateral oophorectomy performed with hysterectomy results in a sudden menopause with rapid onset of menopausal symptoms if performed in a premenopausal woman
	Women who undergo hysterectomy with ovarian conservation have a higher chance of premature menopause. It may be that the ovarian blood supply is affected by the procedure
Autoimmune	Autoimmune disorders of the thyroid, adrenal and pancreas are associated with POF
Radiation	Gonadotoxicity can occur with doses of radiation as low as 5–20 Gy. These doses are commonly used in standard radiotherapy regimes and there is a dose-related effect. The effect can be permanent or temporary
Chemical toxins	The ovary is sensitive to the effects of chemotherapy and the damage can be temporary or permanent. The effect is related to the dose received and the length of treatment
	Smokers have an earlier menopause than non-smokers; polycyclic aromatic hydrocarbons, which are found in high quantities in cigarette smoke, have ovaritoxic effects
Infection	Mumps is occasionally associated with POF

with a low oestradiol level. This should be repeated at least once to confirm the diagnosis as high gonadotrophin levels can be seen during ovulation. In a young woman with menopausal symptoms, who continues to menstruate, a normal hormone profile may simply reflect a perimenopausal state. If the history of menopausal symptoms is convincing, repeat blood sampling may be useful.

> Diagnosis of premature ovarian failure is based on at least two incidences where follicle-stimulating hormone level >30 mIU/ml

Menopausal symptoms can often take longer to be recognized as such in a woman who undergoes a premature menopause and this can be a source of much anxiety and confusion. Appropriate initial investigations are described in Table 3.2.

Psychological effects

The implications of premature menopause to the individual woman will depend on her age and circumstances. A 38-year-old who has completed her family and undergoes a pelvic clearance because of severe endometriosis will be more likely to view her loss of ovarian function as a positive event than a 28-year-old nulliparous woman who has a premature menopause because of chemotherapy.

The physical experience of premature menopause has similar implications to a normal menopause in that it means loss of menstruation and fertility, but the psychosocial effects are more complex. Menopause at the age of 50 is perceived as a natural event, within the normal life experience. A premature menopause

Table 3.2
Initial investigation of a woman with an apparent premature menopause

- Serum FSH, luteinizing hormone (LH), oestradiol and prolactin
- Chromosomal analysis
- Autoimmune screen (thyroid function, fasting glucose, renal function, calcium and vitamin B12 levels)
- Pelvic ultrasound

is outwith the 'normal' life experience and can imply a premature ageing process. Premature menopause tends not to be discussed in public or reported widely by the media.

When the menopause occurs early, it can deny women the potential of fertility, which can be experienced as a significant loss, even by women who do not plan further reproduction. For nulliparous women, particularly those who delayed childbearing because of career plans or other circumstances, a premature menopause can result in feelings of regret, guilt and anger which can be directed towards themselves or others. For some women, the opportunity to express these feelings openly can help them to deal with the diagnosis.

Women faced with a diagnosis of premature menopause can experience feelings of isolation. Relationships can be adversely affected, and it may be that formal counselling can be of benefit. Support groups can allow women to meet others with a similar experience.

> A premature menopause can have complex psychological effects

Osteoporosis

A premature menopause exposes women to a greater number of years without oestrogens. Bone mineral density decreases gradually after the age of 30 years but the rate of loss accelerates in the years following the onset of menopause (see Chapter 6). Therefore, women with a premature menopause reach a threshold where they are at risk of fracture at an earlier age and, as bone density declines with age, this increased risk will persist throughout their lives if hormone replacement therapy (HRT) is not considered.

Cardiovascular disease

The risk of cardiovascular disease is higher among women who have undergone a premature menopause (see Chapter 7). This effect is most striking in woman with a surgical menopause.

Women with a premature menopause are at greater risk of osteoporosis and cardiovascular disease

Fertility

Assessment by fertility specialists at an appropriate stage allows women to obtain realistic advice regarding their chance of having a child. Conversely, the menopause is rarely a sudden event and spontaneous ovulations are likely during the 'perimenopause'. Those women not desiring fertility therefore require contraception.

A premature menopause can sometimes be anticipated, usually when a malignancy is diagnosed requiring cytotoxic medication or radiotherapy. Gonadotoxicity can be predicted at doses of radiotherapy as low as 5–20 Gy, or 5–20 g of cyclophosphamide; older women are more likely to experience POF for a given dose of radiation. This knowledge may provide an opportunity for conservation of reproductive potential.

Anticipation of a premature menopause may provide the opportunity for conservation of reproductive potential

Gonadal cryopreservation

Freezing of embryos is well established within assisted conception techniques and some women may be able to consider this as an option. It is a time-consuming process, which may not be feasible for patients awaiting treatment for a malignancy. The procedure involves superovulation and oocyte retrieval, and a male partner is required. There have been reports of pregnancies occurring after direct freezing of oocytes. However, this technique remains experimental with few oocytes surviving the freezing and thawing process intact. Future development of a reliable technique of oocyte preservation may allow preservation of fertility for women who are known to be at risk of developing a premature menopause.

Ovum or embryo donation

Compared to sperm donation, oocyte donation is a relatively invasive process that requires a well-motivated altruistic donor, as no payment is allowed. Many women must wait for several years for oocytes donated by a volunteer; alternatively, they may have a personal contact who is willing to assist them. As an alternative to oocyte donation, some couples opt to use embryos created within the course of assisted conception treatment and donated by another couple, as they are surplus to requirements.

The pregnancy rates achieved with donor oocytes are often better than would be expected from the average success rates of *in-vitro* fertilization. Fertility rates and IVF success rates decline significantly for women in their late 30s and early 40s. However, when donor oocytes are used, older recipients have a better chance of conception than would be expected. This presumably reflects the fact that oocyte function declines with age. There is a slightly higher rate of miscarriage with a donor pregnancy and a theoretical concern that there may be potential adverse effects, as the mother has made no genetic contribution to the pregnancy.

Hormone replacement therapy

Hormone replacement therapy (HRT) is the cornerstone of the management of women with a premature menopause. This may be administered using the combined oral contraceptive pill if preferred. Many young women will find this more acceptable than HRT. Although a rare event, it is possible for ovarian function to recover in some cases. The combined pill will provide HRT and contraception if fertility is unwanted.

The prescription of HRT is, essentially, the same as for the woman of average age at menopause. The choice of HRT regime (see Chapter 5) depends on whether the woman has a uterus and what her preference is for route of administration. It is likely that younger women, particularly those who have undergone a sudden surgical menopause, will require higher doses of oestrogen to adequately control symptoms.

The long-term health effects of a premature menopause need to be evaluated together with the patient's other risk factors for osteoporosis and cardiovascular disease. By giving HRT until the average age of menopause, it is hoped that these risks can be reduced to a background level.

Symptom control can be particularly important in younger women with a sudden menopause

Further reading

Anasti JN. Premature ovarian failure: an update. *Fertil Steril* 1998; **70**: 1–15.

Bath LE, Wallace HB, Critchley HO. Late effects of the treatment of childhood cancer on the female reproductive system and the potential for fertility preservation. *Br J Obstet Gynaecol* 2002; **109**: 107–14.

Conway GS, Kaltsas G, Patel A *et al*. Characterisation of idiopathic premature ovarian failure. *Fertil Steril* 1996; **65**: 337–41.

Donnez J, Godin PA, Qu J *et al*. Gonadal cryopreservation in the young patient with gynaecological malignancy. *Curr Opin Obstet Gynaecol* 2000; **12**: 1–9.

Singer D. A qualitative study of women's experiences. Premature menopause, a multidisciplinary approach. London: Whurr Publishers, 2000: 57–78.

4. Hormone replacement therapy: preparations and routes of administration

The menopause consultation
Preparations
Oestrogens
Progestogens
Selective oestrogen receptor
    modulators
Alternatives to HRT

The menopause consultation

(see flowchart on inside front cover)

Identify symptoms

A menopause consultation can be varied in source. Most women will seek medical attention if menopausal symptoms are problematic; however, others may persevere and only direct questioning will elicit menopausal symptomatology. It is useful to identify which problems are present and their severity. It can be helpful to provide the patient with a written questionnaire such as the modified Greene's Menopause Scale (Figure 4.1). This exercise provides a record that can be used to monitor treatment effects. Expectations of hormone replacement therapy (HRT) are sometimes over optimistic, eg a women may be disappointed that HRT has not treated her joint discomfort even although it has fully resolved her flushes. An accurate record allows the clinician to understand the woman's expectations and to discuss which symptoms are most likely to be improved by HRT.

Risk:benefit ratio

A consultation for HRT requires an individual assessment of risks and benefits. It is also an opportunity to assess general health status and modify risk factors if possible. Advice about dietary calcium and weight-bearing exercise is particularly important to the menopausal woman. If there is a personal or family history indicating a contraindication to HRT (see Chapter 5), then consideration of alternative options or referral for specialist advice is appropriate. The British Menopause Society has produced a care plan which summarizes a management plan for those in primary care and a handbook outlining management of women with risk factors.

Investigations

As discussed in Chapter 2, hormone levels are rarely helpful. Routine assessment should include:

- monitoring of blood pressure
- cervical cytology
- mammography.

There is no evidence that routine vaginal or breast examination is helpful. Women who complain of gynaecological symptoms such as heavy, painful or unscheduled bleeding will require vaginal examination and possibly referral. Breast examination is obviously required in the context of breast symptoms.

Prescribing HRT

Assessment of current menstrual status will decide the type of HRT prescribed:

- oestrogen only
- sequential
- continuous combined.

The route of administration will usually be dependent on patient choice unless there are risk factors to consider. The initial dose of HRT should be low for postmenopausal women with the aim of increasing the dose after 3 months if there is inadequate symptom control. For perimenopausal women there is little to be gained by starting with low-dose HRT. Standard doses are likely to be required.

The Greene climacteric scale

Name: .... Date: ....

Number: ....

Please indicate the extent to which you are bothered at the moment by any of these symptoms by placing a tick in the appropriate box.

Symptoms	Not at all	A little	Quite a bit	Extremely	Score 0–3
1. Heart beating quickly or strongly					
2. Feeling tense or nervous					
3. Difficulty in sleeping					
4. Excitable					
5. Attacks of panic					
6. Difficulty in concentrating					
7. Feeling tired or lacking in energy					
8. Loss of interest in most things					
9. Feeling unhappy or depressed					
10. Crying spells					
11. Irritability					
12. Feeling dizzy or faint					
13. Pressure or tightness in head or body					
14. Parts of body feel numb or tingling					
15. Headaches					
16. Muscle and joint pains					
17. Loss of feeling in hands or feet					
18. Breathing difficulties					
19. Hot flushes					
20. Sweating at night					
21. Loss of interest in sex					

Figure 4.1
Greene's Menopause Scale.

> Menstrual status will usually decide the type of HRT prescribed and patient choice will determine the route of administration, unless there are other factors to consider

Follow-up

Follow-up at a 3 month interval will allow adequate time for symptoms and many of the nuisance side-effects to improve (breast tenderness, fluid retention, nausea, see Chapter 5). The exception is erratic vaginal bleeding on continuous combined therapy, which will often improve between 3 and 6 months after commencing therapy. It is helpful to give realistic advice at the outset and offer follow-up to all women. Many side-effects will settle with time but a follow-up appointment should always be given to review problems. A point of contact (ideally a telephone number) for use between the first visit and follow-up can be useful.

Preparations

The range of hormone preparations available for the management of menopausal symptoms increases every year. The sheer number of options can be confusing to both women and their doctors.

HRT can be divided into groups according to the constituents and route of administration:

- **Oestrogen alone:** suitable only for hysterectomized women.
- **Oestrogen + progestogen regimes:** women with a uterus require the addition of progestogen therapy to prevent endometrial hyperplasia (see Chapter 7). Women who have undergone endometrial ablative therapies should also be considered to require progestogen, even if they have experienced a prolonged episode of amenorrhoea following the ablative procedure.
  - Sequential therapy: suitable for peri- and early post-menopausal women. Daily oestrogen is given with 12–14 days of progestogen every month to induce a regular withdrawal bleed. There is a

demonstrable increase in the incidence of endometrial cancer with prolonged use of sequential HRT and continuous combined therapy is likely to represent a safer long-term option.

  - Long cycle therapy: daily oestrogen is given with 14 days of progestogen every 3 months, resulting in a 3-monthly withdrawal bleed. This preparation has been developed as an alternative to sequential therapy with less frequent withdrawal bleeds. The bleeds are often prolonged and heavy, which has limited the widespread use of this preparation.
  - Continuous combined therapy: only suitable for women who are unlikely to have significant endogenous hormone production. Daily oestrogen and progestogen are given with the aim of achieving a no-bleed state. If a woman has been amenorrhoeic for 12 months, she can be commenced directly on continuous combined therapy.

> Continuous combined HRT therapy is likely to represent the safest long-term option for the endometrium of postmenopausal women with a uterus

Vaginal bleeding

The vast majority of postmenopausal women will be bleed-free on continuous combined therapy; however, there is a high incidence of breakthrough bleeding in the first months of use. This usually settles with time if the woman has been appropriately selected.

A woman who is perimenopausal or only recently menopausal tends to have some endogenous hormone production, which can lead to erratic bleeding on continuous combined therapy. Women who are still menstruating and those with an inadequate period of amenorrhoea should initially commence sequential HRT, as the chance of obtaining a bleed-free state on continuous treatment is very low.

Ideally, sequential HRT should be limited to perimenopausal and early menopausal women with the aim of transferring to a continuous combined preparation. The difficult decision is when to transfer to a no-bleed preparation. Most women who have been on HRT for 2 years will have minimal endogenous hormone production; however, some women may have started HRT in the early perimenopausal phase, which often lasts about 4 years.

> Sequential HRT should be limited to perimenopausal and early menopausal women

Oestrogens

Potent synthetic oestrogens, such as ethinyl oestradiol and mestranol, are no longer used in HRT regimes due to their metabolic side-effects. Instead, most of the oestrogens used in HRT preparations occur naturally (Table 4.1). These oestrogens are either synthesized or derived from pregnant mares' urine, yams or soya beans.

Oestradiol is the most potent physiological oestrogen and is available for administration orally, transdermally and vaginally. When given orally, a substantial proportion of oestradiol is metabolized to oestrone during first-pass metabolism in the liver. The doses given in standard HRT result in levels of oestradiol similar to physiological levels but with supra-physiological levels of oestrone. In contrast, transdermal administration gives a more physiological ratio of oestradiol to oestrone.

Oestriol is available for administration orally and vaginally. It is poorly absorbed orally but is absorbed well from the vagina.

Table 4.1
Natural oestrogens used in HRT preparations

Conjugated equine oestrogens
Oestradiol
Oestrone
Oestriol
Oestropipate

Conjugated equine oestrogens (Premarin) contain up to ten different oestrogenic compounds, including oestrone. Worldwide, this potent oral HRT is the most commonly used and most of the randomized controlled trials currently in progress are using conjugated oestrogens. One of its disadvantages is that it is impossible to measure serum levels of conjugated oestrogens within the limits of a standard medical laboratory. It is therefore difficult to investigate absorption in women who have a poor response to therapy.

Routes of administration

The different routes of administration are compared in Table 4.2.

Oral administration

Oral administration was the first method to be used widely and it remains the most commonly used route in the UK. Progestogen can be administered within the same tablet to ensure progestogen compliance.

> Oral administration is the most commonly used route in the UK

After oestrogen is absorbed by the gut, it undergoes first-pass metabolism by the liver. The metabolic effects are greater with oral compared with parenteral administration (Table 4.3), which can be both beneficial and potentially detrimental. In particular, oral HRT has a significant effect on serum lipid levels with a very favourable rise in high-density lipoprotein (HDL) cholesterol levels and a corresponding fall in low-density lipoprotein (LDL) levels. Triglyceride levels, coagulation and fibrinolysis can, however, increase. The implications of this are discussed in Chapter 7.

Oral administration is once daily and a high dose has to be given to maintain adequate levels for 24 hours. Women who experience dose-related side-effects with hormones, eg nausea, breast

Table 4.2
Advantages and disadvantages of different routes of HRT administration.

	Advantages	Disadvantages

Oral	Easy to take
	Cheap
	Wide choice
	Oral progestogen can be
	  co-administered
	Elevates HDL
		Daily dosing
		High dose required
		Variation in absorption
		Poor absorption with gastrointestinal
		  dysfunction/post surgery
		Alters hepatic protein synthesis
		Tablets contain lactose
		May elevate triglycerides

Transdermal	Low-dose pure oestrogen Avoids first-pass metabolic effects Physiological oestradiol:oestrone ratio Reduces triglycerides Progesterone can be co-administered Variable dosing system	More expensive Variation in absorption Skin irritation Less effect on HDL
Subcutaneous implants	Pure oestradiol 6-monthly insertion High blood levels achievable Avoids first-pass metabolic effects Physiological oestradiol/oestrone ratio Can be given with testosterone Compliance guaranteed	Surgical procedure Unable to control absorption Risk of tachyphylaxis Difficult to remove Prolonged duration Progestogen needs to be given separately if uterus intact
Vaginal administration	Very effective for vaginal symptoms Avoids first-pass metabolic effects Lasts for 3 months	Progestogen needs to be given separately if uterus intact Ring can fall out

Nasal administration	Avoids first-pass metabolic effects
	Familiar method of drug administration
	Peak levels of oestradiol achieved
	  rapidly with subsequent low levels
		Progestogen needs to be given
		  separately if uterus intact
		Nasal side-effects occasionally

tenderness or migraine (see Chapter 5), may find that oral preparations are more likely to exacerbate their symptoms. Absorption can also vary and women with malabsorptive problems often benefit from parenteral administration.

Table 4.3
Metabolic effects of oestrogen administered orally and transdermally

Metabolic parameter	Oral administration	Transdermal administration
HDL cholesterol	Increases	Neutral
LDL cholesterol	Decreases	Decreases
Triglyceride	Increases	Neutral
Coagulation	Increases	Neutral
Fibrinolysis	Increases	Neutral
C reactive protein	Increase	Neutral

Transdermal administration

Transdermal preparations include oestradiol gel that is applied twice daily, and a variety of adhesive patches. Patches contain either a reservoir of hormone or the hormone is dissolved in the adhesive, allowing them to last for several days and some for up to a week. Progestogen can be co-administered within a patch, which is an aid to compliance, but not with a gel preparation.

The hormone is released steadily from the patch and systemic levels of oestrogen are similar to physiological values with an oestradiol:oestriol ratio of 1:1.

The transdermal route avoids first-pass metabolism and the metabolic effects are different from oral administration. In particular, coagulation is likely to be less affected than with oral administration (see Table 4.2).

> The transdermal route is likely to have less effect on coagulation than the oral route

Skin irritation and allergic reactions are relatively common with transdermal preparations and the patches can fall off. From a compliance point of view, some women find the weekly, or twice weekly, application of patches a convenient method, whereas others find that they forget to replace their patch and that a daily routine would be easier.

Transdermal absorption can be variable and it may be helpful to measure serum oestradiol levels if a woman has a poor response to therapy with a plan to increase the dose or change the route of administration if inadequate levels are achieved.

Subcutaneous implants

Oestradiol and testosterone can both be administered as a subcutaneous implant which last for 4–6 months. Insertion of these solid crystalline pellets of hormones requires infiltration of local anaesthetic and a 5 mm incision in the abdominal skin. Implants, which are the only method of administration that guarantees compliance, are popular with users and most women who commence implants will continue to use them.

As with other parenteral methods, an implant avoids first-pass metabolism and the oestradiol:oestrone ratio produced is more physiological than that achieved by the oral route.

Some patients, particularly younger women and those who experience mood disorders during the menopause, require slightly higher levels of hormones to achieve symptom control and implants are the optimal way of achieving this.

Most practitioners check circulating oestradiol levels annually, although this is probably unnecessary if 50 mg or less is given at no more than 6-monthly intervals.

One relatively rare complication of implant use is the phenomenon of tachyphylaxis. The woman becomes less responsive to oestradiol implants and requires increasing doses to achieve any kind of symptom control, despite very high serum levels of oestradiol. This phenomenon usually only occurs in women who have taken high doses of oestradiol with no monitoring of serum levels, or in whom implants have been given at more frequent intervals than 6-monthly. There are, however, concerns about the health effects of sustained high levels of oestradiol.

Vaginal administration

The vaginal mucosa absorbs oestradiol well and systemic levels that are adequate to treat vasomotor symptoms can be achieved. Rapid absorption will occur with creams or tablets; however, the levels will not be maintained over an adequate time period. A slow-release vaginal ring has been developed that allows steady release of hormone to the vaginal and systemic tissues. A low-dose version, Estring, minimizes systemic effects but provides excellent treatment of urogenital atrophy. A higher dose ring, Menoring, gives adequate levels to treat systemic symptoms.

As with other parenteral methods of HRT administration, vaginal administration is likely to have less effect on coagulation, fibrinolysis and lipids than treatment by the oral route.

Nasal administration

The nasal mucosa provides an absorptive surface of 160m². Rapid uptake of oestradiol occurs and the resulting pharmacokinetics are very different from other routes of administration. Peak levels are achieved within about 20 minutes of administration and thereafter the levels rapidly decline. However, a daily dose of 300 mg of nasal oestradiol is comparable to

2 mg of oral oestradiol with regard to the treatment of flushes. Nasal application of drugs appears to be well tolerated and avoids first-pass metabolism by the liver.

Progestogens

Progesterone is denatured by oral administration but some progesterone and testosterone derivatives are metabolically active via oral routes (Table 4.4).

Norethisterone and levonorgestrel can be administered via transdermal patches. Vaginal gels containing progesterone are available and licensed for use with HRT. Progestin can be administered into the uterus via the levonorgestrel-secreting intrauterine system (LNG-IUS). The LNG-IUS is not licensed for use as HRT in the UK; however, it is anticipated that a lower dose device with a smaller diameter for ease of insertion and developed specifically for postmenopausal women, will become available.

The derivation of a particular progestogen will contribute to any side-effects experienced, eg androgenic side-effects such as acne (see Chapter 5). These may be improved by changing to an alternative progestogen, eg medroxyprogesterone acetate or dydrogesterone.

Tibolone is a synthetic steroid with oestrogenic, progestogenic and androgenic actions. It can achieve a bleed-free state if used in post-menopausal women. As with continuous combined HRT, irregular bleeding will result if

Table 4.4 Orally active progesterone and testosterone derivatives	
Progesterone derivatives	Dydrogesterone
	Medroxyprogesterone
	Hydroxyprogesterone
Testosterone derivatives	Norethisterone
	Desogestrel
	Norgestimate
	Norgestrel
	Levonorgestrel

used by perimenopausal women. The androgenic effect can also improve libido for some women.

Selective oestrogen receptor modulators

Oestrogens act on many organs and tissues, with both negative and positive effects depending on the target organ. Selective oestrogen receptor modulators (SERMs) have been developed with the aim of maximizing the benefits of oestrogens, in particular the prevention of osteoporosis, while minimizing the risks of stimulation of the breast and endometrium. Raloxifene was the first compound specifically developed as a SERM, but the most familiar is tamoxifen, which is used widely in the treatment of breast cancer.

However, their use as a replacement for oestrogen remains limited as none is effective in the treatment of vasomotor symptoms. Currently, SERMs are used mainly for the management of osteoporosis in the asymptomatic woman.

Alternatives to HRT

The menopause and the perimenopause are the ideal times to assess a woman's long-term health risks and to modify them if possible. Several issues are pertinent to the menopausal woman, including a good diet, exercise and reduction of smoking and alcohol consumption. Many of these fall within the remit of general health promotion but can improve the symptoms of the menopausal transition and have beneficial longterm effects on health. It is often difficult to provide adequate time to explore fully all of these issues along with the potential implications of HRT within the context of a standard consultation. They are perhaps better discussed within a well-woman clinic, where more time can be set aside.

The alternative health options often provide a more holistic approach than is offered by standard medical practice. However, there is a lack of evidence of efficacy of many of these therapies and it is unfortunate if women with significant menopausal symptoms are disillusioned by an expensive alternative option that may have few side-effects but is of minimal benefit.

Herbal remedies include black cohosh (part of the buttercup family), ginseng and dong quai, a Chinese herbal remedy. Dietary supplements, such as vitamin E and evening primrose oil, are also recommended. As yet, there is little trial evidence of benefit from these preparations with regard to menopausal symptoms. There is also little evidence of the safety of these remedies, which are often classified as food supplements and as such are not subject to the same regulations as the pharmaceutical industry.

There is much interest in phytoestrogens, which are derived from plants and have a chemical structure similar to oestrogen. They bind to oestrogen receptors but are biologically much less active than oestrogen and also seem to have an antioestrogen effect. The three main types are:

- isoflavones
- coumestans
- lignans.

The most potent are the isoflavones, found in high quantities in soy and legumes. Small randomized controlled trials have demonstrated a slight reduction in the frequency of vasomotor symptoms when phytoestrogens are compared to placebo.

Isoflavones have been shown to have some positive effects on lipid levels and to lower vascular resistance in postmenopausal women. The US FDA has approved a 25-mg daily dose of soy protein to reduce the risk of heart disease. There is much interest in its potential value in the reduction of breast and other oestrogen-dependent cancers, as differences in the amounts of soy in the diet have been suggested as a reason for the differences in rates of cardiovascular disease and breast cancer between cultures. It may also be that a diet rich in soy-containing foods is responsible for the low incidence of menopausal problems among Japanese women. A community-based study of Japanese women showed that high soy intake is associated with a decrease in menopausal symptoms.

Further reading

Crook D. The metabolic consequences of treating postmenopausal women with non-oral hormone replacement therapy. *Br J Obstet Gynaecol* 1997; **104**: 4–13.

Davis SR. Phytoestrogen therapy for menopausal symptoms? There's no good evidence that it's any better than placebo. *Br Med J* 2001; **323**: 354–5.

Glazier GM, Bowman MA. A review of the evidence for the use of phytoestrogens as a replacement for traditional estrogen replacement therapy. *Arch Intern Med* 2001; **161**: 1161–72.

Khastgir G, Studd J. Patient's outlook, experience, and satisfaction with hysterectomy, bilateral oophorectomy, and subsequent continuation of hormone replacement therapy. *Am J Obstet Gynecol* 2000; **183**: 1427–33.

Kroon UB, Tengborn L, Rita H et al. The effects of transdermal oestradiol and oral progestogens on haemostasis variables. *Br J Obstet Gynaecol* 1997; **104**: 32–7.

Nagata C, Takatsuka N, Kawakami N et al. Soy product intake and hot flashes in Japanese women: results from a community-based prospective study. *Am J Epidemiol* 2001; **153**: 790–7.

Nestel PJ, Yamashita T, Sasahara T et al. Soy isoflavones improve systemic arterial compliance but not plasma lipids in menopausal and perimenopausal women. *Arterio Thromb Vasc Biol* 1997; **17**: 3392–8.

Raudaskoski T, Tapanainen J, Tomas E et al. Intrauterine 10mg and 20mg levonorgestrel systems in postmenopausal women receiving oral oestrogen replacement therapy: clinical, endometrial and metabolic response. *Br J Obstet Gynaecol* 2002; **109**: 136–44.

Rymer JM. The effects of tibolone. *Gynecol Endocrinol* 1998; **12**: 213–20.

Scarabin PY, Alhenc-Gelas M, Plu-Bureau G et al. Effect of oral and transdermal estrogen/progesterone regimens on blood coagulation and fibrinolysis in postmenopausal women: a randomised controlled trial. *Arterio Thromb Vasc Biol* 1997; **17**: 3071–8.

St Germaine A, Peterson CT, Robinson JG et al. Isoflavone-rich or isoflavone-poor soy protein does not reduce menopausal symptoms during 24 weeks of treatment. *Menopause* 2001; **8**: 17–26.

Studd J, Pornel B, Marton I et al. Efficacy and acceptability of intranasal 17 beta-oestradiol for menopausal symptoms: randomised dose-response study. *Lancet* 1999; **353**: 1574–8.

5. Hormone replacement therapy: uptake and suitability

Uptake
Compliance
Side-effects
Contraindications

Increased expectations of physical and mental wellbeing and cultural changes over the past 50 years have significantly affected the lifestyle of women in the developed world; a menopausal woman today may have a very different lifestyle from that of her mother and grandmother. Women are less likely to tolerate symptoms that cause distress or inconvenience, particularly as more of them are employed and holding positions of responsibility at work, having achieved equal status with men. At a crucial point in a woman's career, she may find herself let down by her failing ovaries. HRT offers an opportunity for women to maintain health and wellbeing.

Life expectancy has increased in developed societies and the number of people who experience chronic degenerative diseases in later life has grown. Achieving quality of life in later years is becoming as important as longevity itself. The use of HRT is likely to be associated with a significant reduction in the risk of developing osteoporosis, Alzheimer's disease and cancer of the colon (see Chapters 6 and 8), which cause significant morbidity and mortality for women in later life.

> The use of HRT is probably associated with a reduced risk of osteoporotic fracture, colon cancer and Alzheimer's disease

Uptake

Despite the apparent benefits of HRT with regard to the management of menopausal symptoms and prevention of degenerative disorders associated with the menopause, uptake remains low in the UK (around 30% depending on socioeconomic status) and many women do not even collect their prescription.

> Uptake of HRT remains low in the UK, but the reasons for this are not fully understood

The reasons for the low uptake are poorly understood. It may be that women experience fewer problems with menopausal symptoms than is assumed. Alternatively, women experiencing menopausal symptoms may decline HRT because of fear of the potential side-effects. There remains a degree of pressure placed on women to 'cope' with menopausal symptoms and the need for HRT can be perceived as a hormonal crutch to treat a condition that is a natural life event. There is also a reluctance to commence what is perceived as long-term medication.

For a woman facing the experience of the menopause, the decision of whether or not to take HRT is frequently the subject of much soul-searching and is likely to be affected by external factors. It is entirely appropriate that in an increasingly patient-driven society, this decision rests with the individual woman. She will be guided by careful consideration of her symptoms and what the benefits and disadvantages are likely to be. A woman should be provided with information that is as unbiased as possible and the evidence must be interpreted as best as it can be for the individual patient. This responsibility to give accurate information regarding HRT extends to the media, which in the past may have promoted a public overestimation of the risk of, in particular, breast cancer with HRT usage.

Socioeconomic status

HRT use is associated with:

- a higher socioeconomic status
- hysterectomy
- Caucasian race
- having private medical insurance
- favourable health behaviours, including attending for smears, mammograms and cholesterol checks.

In view of this, it may be that some of the benefits seen for HRT users are due to a 'healthy user bias'.

However, the disparity between users and non-users appears to be less than in the past. The large randomized controlled trials currently underway should clarify the effects of socioeconomic status. An American study examined the changes in hormone use between 1989 and 1996. It showed that HRT use increased from 5.7% in 1989 to 10.9% in 1996. There was some disparity in usage between different groups, with a lower use in non-whites compared to whites and lower use in medicaid patients when compared to those with private insurance. This discrepancy was significantly less obvious in the later years of the study and it does appear that the influence of socioeconomic factors on the use of HRT is declining.

The level of uptake of HRT is related to the amount of information that women have access to and disparity persists. Studies have shown that women with greater years of education and affluence are more likely to obtain information on the menopause. The effectiveness of any health promotion regarding the menopause will be affected by these factors. HRT use and long-term compliance are very high (over 80%) among female gynaecologists. The implication is that this well-informed group could reflect greater use among the general population if the understanding of the benefits and risks were higher.

A survey of 103 perimenopausal female patients within a London general practice assessed perception of future health risks. This showed that women tend to underestimate their risk of cardiovascular disease and overestimate their risk of breast cancer. When asked to re-estimate the risks in association with HRT use they believed that HRT would:

- reduce risk of osteoporosis by about 10%
- increase risk of breast cancer by 8%
- have no effect on cardiovascular risk.

Attitudes of others

The reasons why women choose or decline HRT are complex and are affected by many influences, including the views of those who are most likely to be providing advice regarding the menopause and HRT and who are also supporting the women's decisions. For some women, the attitude of her family doctor is most important, for others the influence of family, friends and colleagues may be just as influential. A negative report of side-effects from another woman is a frequently reported reason for avoiding HRT. Positive accounts can be equally damaging if the woman is inadvertently disappointed when she expected the miraculous change that her friends report – 'I thought I would be a new woman'.

Compliance

Ongoing compliance with HRT can be low, with 25% of patients stopping therapy within 6 months. To improve compliance, several issues have to be addressed and an opportunity must be given for women to ask questions. An honest discussion of the risks and benefits, as understood at present, is required for all women who are prescribed HRT. Fear of cancer is a common reason for declining such treatment and is an important cause of low compliance. This is a highly emotive issue and it is difficult to translate population risks to an individual. The results of the most recently reported study on HRT use, the Women's Health Initiative (WHI), were reported as a:

- 26% increase in the risk of breast cancer
- 29% increase in the risk of coronary heart disease
- 41% increase in the risk of stroke.

The actual numbers of extra events that occurred were 8 extra cases of breast cancer, 7 extra coronary heart disease events and 8 more strokes per 10,000 women using HRT. It is useful to compare other risk factors when considering the implications of HRT use. There is a 3–4 fold increase in the risk of heart disease with cigarette smoking and the burden of obesity continues to increase in developed societies. Women who delay childbirth until after 30 years of age have a two-fold increased risk of developing breast cancer when compared to women who have their first child aged less than 20 years.

> 25% of women stop using HRT within 6 months

The potential side-effects should be explained so that they can be anticipated. As with many therapies, the ability of a patient to tolerate side-effects often depends on the perceived benefits of the therapy. If they are as bad, or worse, than the menopausal symptoms, then the woman is simply exchanging one set of unpleasant symptoms for another and she is therefore less likely to continue with HRT. Older women who are receiving HRT for long-term health reasons, such as osteoporosis, are less likely to tolerate side-effects as they are often asymptomatic. There is an increasing range of options available to suit the individual woman but many women will not return to their doctor if problems develop. It is therefore important to give realistic advice at the outset and offer follow-up to all women. Many side-effects will settle with time but a follow-up appointment should always be given to review problems. A point of contact (ideally, a telephone number) for use between the first visit and follow-up can be useful.

> A follow-up appointment should always be given to review any problems with HRT

Side-effects

Vaginal bleeding

The most common symptom causing compliance problems is continued vaginal bleeding in the form of withdrawal bleeds for women on sequential preparations (see Chapter 4); this is a particular problem for the older woman who has been amenorrhoeic for many years.

> Withdrawal bleeds are the most common symptom causing compliance problems in women taking sequential HRT preparations

The development of continuous combined no-bleed preparations (see Chapter 4) has allowed women who find withdrawal bleeds unacceptable to continue using HRT. However, even with these preparations, a significant minority of women will have continued vaginal bleeding. Usually, this is not heavy but can be present every day. The bleeding improves within the first 6 months for the vast majority, but many will stop HRT before this time. To prevent a high dropout rate, it is important that a woman commencing a continuous combined preparation is counselled that bleeding might be present for several months.

> Women taking continuous combined HRT preparations must be counselled that some bleeding might occur for several months

Changing to another continuous combined preparation after only a few months of use is inadvisable, as the bleeding pattern will often improve within 3–6 months. If bleeding continues beyond 6 months, it is less likely that it will improve without intervention. Investigation may be merited and this is discussed in more detail in Chapter 9.

Altering the dose of oestrogen or progestogen or, alternatively, taking tibolone (a synthetic steroid), can reduce breakthrough bleeding. The use of a levonorgestrel-secreting intrauterine system (LNG-IUS) can allow perimenopausal women to achieve amenorrhoea. The LNG-IUS is licensed for treatment of menorrhagia but, as yet, its use as HRT remains unlicensed in the UK (see Chapter 4).

Weight gain

Weight gain, or concern over potential weight gain, is a frequently cited reason for stopping HRT. Although several studies have shown that weight gain tends to occur in the middle years regardless of whether a woman is taking HRT, many women complain of a subjective sense of gaining weight after they commence HRT. It may be that hormonal effects on tissues, such as the breast, can contribute to this sensation, and these effects tend to settle with use.

> Weight tends to be gained in the middle years regardless of whether a woman is taking HRT or not

Changes do occur in the distribution of adipose tissue following the menopause, with an increase in the proportion of central abdominal fat. This 'android' deposition of fat is associated with a higher risk of cardiovascular disease. The use of HRT causes redistribution of fat to 'female' areas, such as the hips. It is good practice to make a note of the patient's weight at clinic visits so that she may be reassured that she is not in fact gaining large amounts of weight.

Oestrogenic effects

- Breast tenderness
- Nausea
- Leg cramps.

Most of these side-effects will improve with time. If after 3 months the side-effects continue to be problematic, reduction of the dose can be effective. If breast tenderness persists, another option is the addition of gamolenic acid.

Progestogenic effects

Some women are troubled by progestogenic side-effects, including:

- fluid retention and bloating
- breast tenderness
- headache
- acne and greasy skin.

Many of these side-effects will settle with time and a woman, appropriately counselled, is more likely to continue with HRT.

Some women, often those with a history of premenstrual problems, are particularly sensitive to the effects of progestogen. Progestogen intolerance causes most problems for women who are using sequential HRT, with intermittent exposure to progestogen. Changing to a continuous preparation can sometimes improve symptoms.

> Women with a history of premenstrual problems are particularly sensitive to the effects of progestogen

Depending on the pattern of symptoms, a different progestogen can be of benefit, eg if androgenic side-effects (such as hair growth or acne) are present, then a less androgenic preparation can be used. A quarterly regime is available where the patient receives progestogen every 3 months, thus minimizing exposure. The LNG-IUS results in minimal systemic absorption of progestogen and can be used as endometrial protection. Alternatively, vaginally administered progesterone can be used with fewer systemic effects and potential side-effects.

Contraindications

The contraindications to the combined pill were initially used as contraindications to HRT. However, as the doses of hormone used in HRT are now much closer to physiological levels, the list of absolute contraindications has been shortened (Table 5.1). If a woman falls into one of these categories but requires HRT, she should be referred to a specialist menopause clinic where an assessment of the risks can be made with advice from appropriate sources (breast surgeons, physicians, haematologists).

For a woman who has a relative contraindication to HRT use (Table 5.2), an individual assessment of the risks and benefits is required. In some cases this will require specialist referral, particularly where a thrombotic tendency is present.

Referral to a specialist menopause clinic may also be of benefit where women have had continued problems with side-effects or symptom control despite trying different preparations of HRT.

Table 5.1
Absolute contraindications to HRT

- Breast cancer, endometrial cancer or other oestrogen-dependent tumours
- Undiagnosed vaginal bleeding
- Pregnancy or breastfeeding
- Thromboembolic disease or symptomatic thrombophilia
- Severe renal or liver disease
- Acute intermittent porphyria

Table 5.2
Relative contraindications to HRT

Relative contraindications	Family history of thromboembolic disease Otoscerlosis Body mass index >30 kg/m^2 Systemic lupus erythematosus Malignant melanoma
Situations where careful monitoring is required	Severe endometriosis Cholelithiasis Hypertension Diabetes Migraine Epilepsy

HRT use and other medical conditions

The remainder of this chapter will briefly examine the role of HRT in various medical conditions. Osteoporosis, venous thromboembolic disease and cardiovascular disease are also discussed in Chapters 6, 7 and 8; HRT and malignancy is discussed in Chapter 9.

Dementia

Dementia is a heterogeneous disorder present in 10% of the population over the age of 65 years and 50% of the population over the age of 85 years. Alzheimer's disease is the most common cause of dementia and there are few therapeutic options for this disorder. Women appear to be more at risk of developing Alzheimer's disease than men and prospective cohort studies have shown that oestrogen use is associated with a 50% reduction in risk. It maybe that oestrogen has a role in the prevention of Alzheimer's disease and this could account for the lower rates of the disease in HRT users. Unfortunately, randomized controlled trials of the effect of oestrogen on the cognitive abilities of women with dementia have failed to show an improvement.

Systemic lupus erythematosus

There is a theoretical concern that the use of HRT can increase disease activity for women with systemic lupus erythematosus (SLE). There is little hard evidence that this is the case and women with SLE have a higher risk of osteoporosis due to corticosteroid use. It is wise to consult the patient's rheumatologist before starting HRT. For women with SLE with anti-phospholipid antibodies the risk of thrombosis is increased and HRT should be used with significant caution. Referral to a specialist clinic would be required.

Endometriosis

Endometriosis is a hormone-sensitive disease, which responds well to a hypoestrogenic state. For the majority of women, the low levels of oestrogen provided by HRT are insufficient to stimulate development of endometriosis. In women with severe endometriosis, implants should be avoided and some practitioners would delay starting HRT for 6 months after hysterectomy. There is no good evidence that this is required and women with endometriosis are often at an increased risk of osteoporosis because of medical therapies and early bilateral oophorectomy.

Otosclerosis

Otoclerosis is an inherited condition causing progressive deafness that can be accelerated by pregnancy and oral contraceptives. There is no evidence that the use of HRT has a detrimental effect but the condition is likely to progress with age.

Epilepsy

Some anticonvulsants can induce liver enzymes. In view of this, a transdermal route may be preferable to an oral route of HRT delivery; however, little data exists.

Hypertension

Usually HRT does not increase blood pressure but it can on rare occasions. it is good practice to monitor blood pressure 3 monthly for the first 6 months after starting HRT and yearly thereafter. There is no contraindication to HRT use in women with controlled hypertension.

Migraine

Migraine can occasionally be exacerbated by HRT (see Chapter 2). There is no evidence that HRT use increases the risk of stroke for women who suffer from migraine. A low-dose transdermal preparation provides more stable oestrogen levels and most women will notice an improvement in symptoms. Occasionally the sequential progestogen component provides the trigger for migraine. In this instance, change to continuous combined if feasible or use a route that minimizes systemic progestogen absorption (such as vaginal or intrauterine).

Stroke

The relationship between HRT and stroke is far from clear. Some studies have shown a reduced risk for HRT users, most have shown little effect and a few have suggested an increased risk. These differences between studies may, in part, be methodological. Most studies did not define which stroke subtypes occurred in their populations. Cerebrovascular disease is a heterogeneous entity which may arise from a wide variety of pathophysiological processes. Approximately 85% of strokes are ischaemic in origin with 10% caused by haemorrhage. At least one-quarter of all ischaemic strokes are caused by emboli that have arisen from another source. Such emboli may arise from a variety of sites, including the venous circulation with paradoxical embolization through a right-to-left shunt. Between 40–50% of young patients with stroke have been shown to have a patent foramen ovale, which may allow passage of venous clot into the arterial tree.

There does appear to be a relationship between higher levels of sex steroids and stroke. There is a small increase in the risk of stroke during pregnancy and whilst using the contraceptive pill. This is a dose-related effect, with low-dose combined pills (30 micrograms or less) having only a very minor affect on stroke risk – but this risk increases significantly when the dose is 50 micrograms or more.

The WHI, the first large placebo-controlled trial of HRT in healthy women, showed an increased risk of stroke among HRT users. The absolute numbers of patients were small; 127 strokes among the 8506 women on HRT and 85 strokes among the 8102 women on placebo. As yet information has not been published on stroke subtypes and a potential mechanism for an increased risk of stroke remains unclear. There is no evidence that oestrogen prevents recurrent stroke. A placebo-controlled trial of 2.8 years of oral oestradiol in 664 women with a recent ischaemic cerebral event showed no evidence of a beneficial effect. There was a higher risk of fatal stroke in the oestradiol group. If a women has had a cerebrovascular event and wishes to use HRT for symptom control she should be referred to a specialist clinic. It may be that a thrombophilia screen is merited, and if HRT is required, a low-dose transdermal preparation would minimize the procoagulant effect of HRT.

Diabetes

Diabetes mellitus is one of the commonest diseases in the westen world and the incidence is increasing rapidly. This is particularly true of type 2 diabetes, which also increases with age. There has been a reluctance to prescribe HRT to women with diabetes, mainly because there is concern that it will impact adversely on carbohydrate metabolism, thus worsening the diabetes.

The most common cause of death in women with diabetes is coronary heart disease. The most likely reason for this is the associated metabolic syndrome which includes hyperlipidaemia, hypertriglyceridaemia, insulin resistance, abnormalities of vascular reactivity and an increase in the likelihood of having a thrombotic event. Although these can be reversed to an extent by good control of the diabetes, cardiovascular disease tends to progress.

In type 1 diabetes, there is no pre-menopausal protection from heart disease as there is in women without diabetes. The reasons for this are unknown. It is thus less clear as to whether HRT might possibly have a place in altering any of these processes. Approximately 20% of the women in the HERS study were diabetics and it was not possible to demonstrate a decreased incidence of heart disease in this group. Reasons for this are summarized in the chapter on cardiovascular disease.

There have been a number of placebo-controlled trials looking at the effect of various HRT regimens in women with diabetes. It would appear that there is no adverse impact of oestrogen replacement on glucose homeostasis. Also, it has been shown that the small doses of progestogen used in HRT do not increase insulin resistance in women with type 2 diabetes. The current recommendation is that transdermal oestrogen is preferred to oral because it does not lead to an increase in triglyceride levels and it has no effect on carbohydrate metabolism. However, there are now some data to suggest that the levels of glycosylated haemoglobin are less in those using oral preparations. Women with diabetes should not be denied HRT because of inappropriate conclusions drawn from studies with the oral contraceptive pill.

Further reading

Ameriso SF, Sahai S. Mechanisms of ischaemia in *in-situ* vascular occlusive disease. Primer on cerebrovascular diseases. San Diego: Academic Press 1997, 279–85.

Chang CL, Donaghy M, Poulter NR. Migraine and stroke in young women. The World Health Organisation Collaborative Study of Cardiovascular Disease and Steroid Hormone Contraception. *BMJ* 1999; **318**: 13–18.

Crawford SL, Casey VA, Avis NE *et al*. A longitudinal study of weight and the menopause transition: results from the Massachusetts Women's Health Study. *Menopause* 2000; **7**: 96–104.

Ettinger B, Pressman A, Silver P. Effect of age on reasons for initiation and discontinuation of hormone replacement therapy. *J North Am Menopause Soc* 1999; **6**: 282–9.

Fisher WA, Sand M, Lewis W *et al*. Canadian menopause study-I: Understanding women's intention to utilise hormone replacement therapy. *Maturitas* 2000; **37**: 1–14.

Hunter M, O'Dea I. Perception of future health risks in mid aged women: estimates with and without behavioural changes and hormone replacement therapy. *Maturitas* 1999; **33**: 37–43.

Isaacs AJ, Britton AR, Mcpherson K. Why do doctors in the UK take hormone replacement therapy? *J Epidemiol Comm Health* 1997; **51**: 373–7.

Kawas C, Resnick S, Morrison A *et al*. A prospective study of estrogen replacement therapy and the risk of developing Alzheimer's: the Baltimore Longitudinal Study of Ageing. *Neurology* 1997; **48**: 1517–21.

Lahita RG. The role of sex hormones in systemic lupus erythematosus. *Curr Opin Rheumatol* 1999; **11**: 352–6.

MacLennan AH, Wilson DH, Taylor AW. Hormone replacement therapy: prevalence, compliance and the 'healthy women' notion. *Climacteric* 1998; **1**: 42–9.

McKinlay JB, McKinlay SJ, Brambilla DJ. Health status and utilisation behaviour associated with menopause. *Am J Epidemiol* 1987; **125**: 110–21.

McNagny SE, Wenger NK, Frank E. Personal use of postmenopausal hormone replacement therapy by women physicians in the United States. *Ann Intern Med* 1997; **127**: 1093–109.

Mulnard RA, Cotman CW, Kawas C et al. Estrogen replacement therapy for treatment of mild to moderate Alzheimer's disease: a randomised controlled trial. *JAMA* 2000; **283**: 1007–15.

Norman RR, Flight IH, Rees MC. Oestrogen and progestogen hormone replacement therapy for perimenopausal and postmenopausal women: weight and body fat distribution (Cochrane Review). Cochrane Library, Issue 2, 2002. Oxford: Update Software

Paganini-Hill A, Henderson VW. Estrogen deficiency and risk of Alzheimer's disease in women. *Am J Epidemiol* 1994; **140**: 256–61.

Stafford RS, Saglam D, Causino N et al. The declining impact of race and insurance status on hormone replacement therapy. *J North Am Menopause Soc* 1998; **5**: 140–4.

Tang MX, Jacobs D, Stern Y et al. Effect of oestrogen during menopause on risk and age of onset of Alzheimer's disease. *Lancet* 1996; **348**: 429–32.

Viscoli CM, Brass LM, Kernan WN et al. A clinical trial of estrogen-replacement therapy after ischaemic stroke. *N Engl J Med* 2001; **345**: 1243–9.

Wang PN, Liao SQ, Liu RS et al. Estrogen for Alzheimer's disease in women. *Neurology* 2000; **54**: 2061–6.

Writing group for the Women's Health Initiative. Risks and benefits of estrogen plus progestin in healthy postmenopausal women. *JAMA* 2002; **288**: 321–33.

6. Osteoporosis

Pathogenesis
Risk factors
Diagnosis
Screening and prevention
Treatment

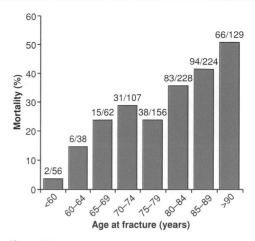

Figure 6.1
Mortality 1 year after proximal femoral fracture in relation to age. (Reproduced with permission from Keene GS, Parker MJ, Pryor GA. Mortality and morbidity after hip fractures. *Br Med J* 1993; **307**: 1248–50.)

The implications of osteoporosis, both to society and to the individual, are considerable. One in three women and one in 12 men will develop osteoporosis. It is estimated that three million patients in the UK have osteoporosis. This translates to over 200,000 fractures annually. About 50% of all patients who experience a fractured hip will lose the ability to live independently and one-third will die within one year (Figure 6.1). The costs to the NHS and Government are currently £1.7 billion per year. The incidence of osteoporosis-related fracture within developed populations has been climbing and this trend is likely to continue. As bone density declines with age, it is likely that increased life expectancy is responsible for most of this increase but it may be that lifestyle changes are also contributing.

> About one-half of patients who fracture their hip lose their ability to live independently and one-third die within a year

Pathogenesis

Bone is formed by the production of an organic matrix (mainly type I collagen), which is then mineralized. It is constantly being removed and replaced in a complex process that is poorly understood. Bone formation appears to be stimulated by bone resorption, as the two processes are normally closely linked. Osteoclastic cells and osteoblastic cells work as

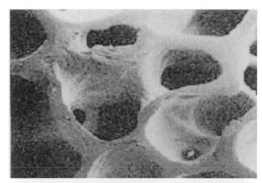
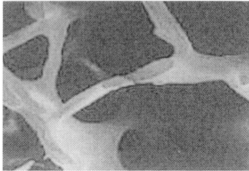

Figure 6.2
Scanning electron micrographs of normal (left) and osteoporotic (right) bone. (Reproduced with permission from Stephen AB, Wallace WA. *J Bone Joint Surg (Br)* 2001; **83**: 316–23.)

a unit, respectively resorbing and reforming bone. In normal bone, these processes are in balance, but in osteoporotic bone, the rate of resorption exceeds that of reforming (Figure 6.2). This process is influenced by many factors including those that maintain calcium homeostasis (Table 6.1).

The World Health Organization defines osteoporosis as a 'progressive systemic skeletal disease characterized by a low bone mass and microarchitectural deterioration of bone tissue, with a consequent increase in bone fragility and susceptibility to fracture'. Bone mass is decreased but is of normal composition: there are fewer trabeculae and thinning of cortical bone but the existing bone is fully mineralized.

Osteoporotic fractures typically occur in sites where there is a high proportion of trabecular bone (Table 6.2), the commonest sites being vertebral bodies and the ends of long bones, in particular the hip and wrist (Figure 6.3).

Table 6.2
Sites at risk of osteoporotic fractures

- Vertebral bodies
- Proximal femur
- Distal radius (Colles' fracture)

Risk factors

Osteoporosis is a multifactorial disorder and whether an individual develops the disease depends on peak bone mass and the rate of its subsequent loss (Table 6.3). Peak bone mass is achieved by about the age of 30 years and bone loss occurs gradually thereafter. It depends on interaction between:

- genetic factors
- nutritional state
- body build
- smoking

Table 6.1
Factors that influence bone remodelling.

Parathyroid hormone	Mobilizes calcium from bone
	Increases urinary phosphate excretion
	Stimulates osteoclasts
	Increases formation of 1,25-dihyroxycholecalciferol
Calcitonin	Reduces number and activity of osteoclasts
	Increases urinary calcium excretion
1,25 dihydroxyvitamin D	Increases calcium absorption from intestine. Increases number of osteoclasts and activity
Oestrogens	Complex effects, stimulate osteoblasts
Fluoride	Stimulates osteoblasts
Glucocorticoids	Inhibit cellular replication and protein synthesis
	Inhibit function of osteoblasts
	Reduce intestinal absorption of calcium and vitamin D
Growth hormone	Increases urinary calcium excretion
	Even greater intestinal absorption of calcium

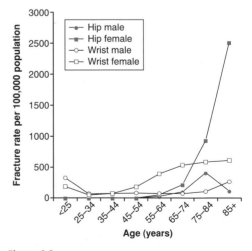

Figure 6.3
Hip and wrist fracture rates by age in men and women.
(Reproduced with permission from Donaldson LJ, Cook A. Incidence of fractures in a geographically defined population. *J Epidemiol Comm Health* 1991; **44**: 241–5.)

- alcohol consumption
- weight-bearing exercise.

In women, the peak bone mass is less than in men and there is an increased rate of loss in the 10 years after the menopause (up to 15% of the skeleton can be lost in these succeeding years). Women have a longer life-expectancy than men and together these factors account for the female preponderance of the disease.

> 15% of a woman's skeleton can be lost in the years following the menopause

Diagnosis

This chapter concentrates on age and menopause-related osteoporosis. However, Table 6.3 serves to illustrate the associated disorders that should be considered. The differential diagnosis of osteoporosis includes:

- multiple myeloma
- metastatic carcinoma
- osteomalacia
- hyperparathyroidism
- osteogenesis imperfecta.

Osteoporosis is a clinically silent condition, which is often diagnosed only after a fracture occurs. There are several techniques for identifying the disease before this stage is reached.

> Osteoporosis is often diagnosed only after fracture occurs

The Royal College of Physicians recommends that the following investigations should be performed:

- full blood count and erythrocyte sedimentation rate
- bone and liver function tests
- renal function tests
- serum thyroid-stimulating hormone.

Table 6.3
Risk factors for osteoporosis

Endocrine	Premature menopause, including hysterectomy or oophorectomy Prolonged amenorrhoea, including exercise-induced and contraceptive methods (eg Depo-Provera) Testosterone deficiency in young men Cushing's syndrome (either spontaneous or iatrogenic) Thyrotoxicosis Hypopituitarism
Nutritional	Anorexia nervosa Starvation Coeliac disease
Genetic	Osteogenesis imperfecta Familial and racial
Lifestyle	Smoking Alcohol
Idiopathic	Juvenile osteoporosis Osteoporosis in young adults
Other	Mastocytosis Longterm heparin administration Cytotoxic therapy Systemic disease, including renal or liver failure

[Adapted from Weatherall DJ, Ledingham JGG, Warrell DA (eds). *Oxford Textbook of Medicine, 3rd edn*. Oxford: Oxford University Press, 1996: 3067]

If indicated, the Royal College of Physicians recommends that the following should also be performed:

- lateral thoracic and lumbar spine X-rays
- serum paraproteins and urine Bence Jones protein
- isotope bone scan
- serum follicle-stimulating hormone (FSH) if the hormonal status is unclear.

Plain X-ray

A plain X-ray will only detect osteoporosis if one-third of bone mass has been lost. Alone, it is of little use as a screening tool, but it is essential in the diagnosis of fractures and to assess vertebral deformity. However, it has been repeatedly shown that even the majority of patients diagnosed with fragility-type fractures are not offered investigation or management of osteoporosis.

Computed tomography and ultrasound

Quantitative computed tomography allows differential measurement of cortical and trabecular bone, but the radiation dose is much higher and the equipment is expensive.

Broadband ultrasound is useful to assess the os calcis, tibia and patella. It has the advantages of being radiation free, relatively cheap, and potentially more portable than dual energy X-ray absorptiometry (DEXA) scanning (see below). The ability of ultrasound to predict fracture risk accurately remains unproven; however, several studies have shown that quantitative ultrasound is better at detecting low bone mass than consideration of clinical risk factors.

It may be that ultrasound should be considered for use as a screening tool before referral for DEXA. A study in Aberdeen, UK, screened 1000 perimenopausal women using both DEXA and broadband ultrasound. Although very few fractures (18 in 17 women) occurred in the 2 years of follow up and the accuracy of prediction was weak, both techniques were comparable in fracture prediction.

Biochemical markers

Serum markers of bone formation are bone-specific alkaline phosphatase and osteocalcin. Markers of bone resorption are the collagen cross-linked deoxypyridinoline and N-telopeptide. These markers correlate well with increased bone turnover such as occurs in the years after the menopause, but their use is mainly limited to clinical trials.

Absorptiometry

Standard techniques used to assess bone density employ photons, which require source renewal, or X-rays, which do not. A single source is used to assess the bone density of appendicular sites, such as the forearm, and

dual energy to assess both appendicular sites and the more clinically relevant axial sites, including the spine and hip.

The most widely used technique is DEXA (Figure 6.4), which has high reproducibility and low radiation doses. DEXA is the gold standard technique for assessment of bone mineral density (BMD) (Figure 6.5). However, availability of DEXA within many parts of the UK would not meet current screening recommendations described by the Royal College of Physicians (see below).

Densitometry techniques do have limitations; measurement can be affected by:

- extraskeletal calcification
- osteophytes
- scoliosis
- vertebral deformity.

Densitometry can also be used to monitor treatment and the spine is considered to be the optimal site for this. Usually, it is not required in women on hormone replacement therapy (HRT), but may be justified for those with malabsorption or on corticosteroid therapy. Other therapies should be monitored as the long-term effects are less well established.

Screening and prevention

Bone mineral density (BMD) is expressed as a standard deviation score in relation to a reference range.

- young adult values – T score (see Table 6.4)
- sex and age-matched values – Z score.

Although it would seem logical to compare a patient to others of the same age and sex, if the Z score is used, then the diagnosis of osteoporosis would not increase with age and it is well established that osteoporosis-related fracture rates increase with age.

Reduced BMD correlates well with increased risk of fracture but BMD cannot accurately identify

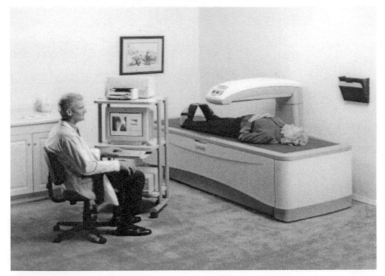

Figure 6.4
DEXA being performed (courtesy of the National Osteoporosis Society).

individuals who will have a fracture. There is significant overlap between the BMDs of those who fracture and those who do not. The number of false positives is only 15% but the number of false negatives is 50%. This means that half of all fractures will occur in women said not to have osteoporosis. In view of this, BMD cannot be recommended as a population screening tool but it has been adopted for selective case screening.

> BMD should be offered to women with risk factors for osteoporosis

The Royal College of Physicians recommends that people in the following groups be offered BMD measurements:

- radiographic evidence of osteopenia and/or vertebral deformity

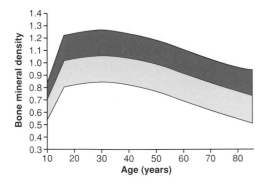

Figure 6.5
Bone mineral density by DEXA. (From: Smith R. Disorders of the skeleton. In: Weatherall DJ, Ledingham JGG, Warrell DA, eds. *Oxford Textbook of Medicine*, 3rd edn. Oxford: Oxford University Press, 1996: 3066.)

Table 6.4
Bone mineral density (BMD) T score

State of bones	T score
Normal	BMD within 1 SD of young adult mean
Osteopenia	BMD between 1 and 2.5 SDs below the young adult mean
Osteoporosis	BMD 2.5 or more SDs below the young adult mean
Severe osteoporosis	BMD 2.5 or more SDs below the young adult mean and there is one or more fracture present

SD, standard deviation

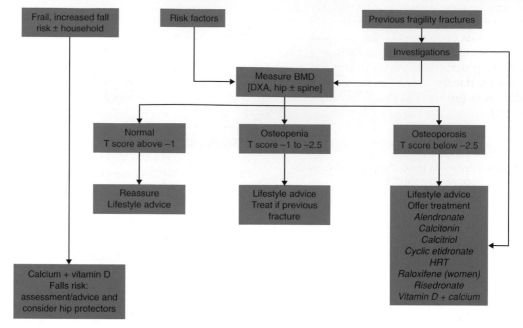

Figure 6.6
Royal College of Physicians' guidelines for the management of osteoporosis.

- loss of height, thoracic kyphosis (after radiographic confirmation of vertebral deformity)
- previous fragility fracture
- prolonged corticosteroid therapy (prednisolone >7.5 mg daily for 6 months or more)
- premature menopause (age <45 years)
- prolonged secondary amenorrhoea (>1 year)
- primary hypogonadism
- chronic disorders associated with osteoporosis
- maternal history of hip fracture
- low body mass index (<19 kg/m^2).

If osteoporosis is identified from assessment of BMD, treatment can be provided to reduce the risk of the individual developing a fracture. As the T score compares a person's BMD to that of the young adult mean, a significant proportion of the elderly will inevitably be shown to be osteopenic. The higher threshold of osteopenia is of clinical relevance in that these patients,

and particularly women who have yet to experience the menopause, should be considered for prevention of further bone loss.

Population-based strategies for the prevention of osteoporosis advise increased physical activity, particularly weight-bearing exercise, reduced smoking and corrected dietary calcium intake. These strategies form part of most health promotion messages and are, undoubtedly, commendable but the evidence that changing lifestyle translates to a reduced risk of fracture is scanty. Only modest increases in BMD have been detected if adults undertake regular weight-bearing exercise. However, it may be that exercise and nutrition are more important in the development of the skeleton in childhood and adolescence and that benefits obtained during the formative years persist until adult life.

Treatment

Guidelines for the management of osteoporosis are summarized in Figure 6.6.

Therapy for prevention of osteoporosis is mainly directed at slowing the accelerated loss of bone mass that occurs in the postmenopausal period. On this basis, a perimenopausal woman with a BMD of between 1 and 2.5 standard deviations below the young adult mean (osteopenia) should be considered for HRT.

> A woman with a bone mineral density 1–2.5 standard deviations below the young adult mean should be considered for HRT

Ideally, treatment will be adjusted to the individual and will depend, to a degree, on the likely cause. Reversible factors, such as smoking, excessive alcohol intake or lack of weight-bearing exercise, should be addressed if possible, as well as factors that may increase the risk of falls, eg sedative medication or an unsafe environment. In patients prone to falls, simple measures such as hip protectors may be helpful.

Calcium and vitamin D

To prevent bone loss an average daily intake of 700 mg of calcium is required. Good dietary sources of calcium are:

- milk and dairy products
- green leafy vegetables
- fish.

Calcium supplementation has a positive effect on BMD in postmenopausal women. The daily dose required to treat osteoporotic bone loss (1000–1500 mg) is significantly higher than the average dietary calcium intake. Dietary manipulation or supplementation should be considered as a preventative measure in menopausal women and as part of treatment of established osteoporosis. Calcium is well tolerated and requires little monitoring.

> 1000–1500 mg daily of calcium is required to treat osteoporotic bone loss

There is evidence for a reduced fracture risk with calcium supplementation, particularly in the elderly. The largest study of 3270 women showed a 26% reduction in non-vertebral fractures in patients who were given daily calcium supplementation together with vitamin D. However, this study was performed on nursing home residents who would be more likely to be calcium and, in particular, vitamin D deficient. Vitamin D supplementation is relevant in elderly housebound patients where exposure to sunlight is minimal; however, there is no evidence that it is of use in community populations.

Oestrogen

Epidemiological evidence suggests that women who experience less exposure to endogenous oestrogen have a higher risk of osteoporosis. Women who undergo a premature menopause have a higher risk of osteoporosis and fracture when compared to women who undergo the menopause at an average age. A low level of endogenous oestradiol in postmenopausal women is associated with a higher risk of fracture (after adjusting for height and weight). Endogenous oestrogen levels are responsible for the relationship between low body mass and risk of osteoporosis. There are higher endogenous levels of oestrogens in obese women because of peripheral aromatization of androgens.

The mechanism of oestrogen's protective effect on bone is not fully understood, but there is evidence for oestrogen receptor sites in osteoblasts and inhibition of cytokine-induced bone resorption.

Some of the earliest evidence of a protective effect of oestrogen on bone was derived from case-control studies. It became apparent that women who experienced fragility fractures were less likely to be HRT users when compared to control groups. The largest of these, a study of 2086 women with hip fractures and 3552 controls, demonstrated a relative risk of 0.55 for hip fracture in women taking oestrogen.

Prospective cohort studies of fracture risk have also demonstrated a strongly protective effect of HRT use. The Framingham study examined 2873 women and found that the relative risk of hip fracture was 0.65 in women who had never used HRT and 0.34 in women who had used HRT in the previous 2 years.

> HRT users are at a significantly reduced risk of osteoporotic fracture

The observational data are persuasive; however, it may be that women who take HRT differ from women who do not. In particular, HRT users may have other positive health behaviours, such as more weight-bearing exercise or higher calcium intake.

The number of randomized controlled trials of the effect of oestrogen on osteoporosis and, particularly, fracture risk is small despite the well-established relationship. Most women decide whether or not to use HRT because of menopausal symptoms. It may be that this leads to difficulty in randomizing large numbers of women to placebo in long-term trials.

One study compared the effects of mestranol and placebo on bone densitometry over a 5-year follow-up in women who had undergone oophorectomy. A significant reduction in height occurred in the placebo group but not the mestranol-treated group. Another study compared the effect of transdermal oestrogen with placebo in 75 women with well-established postmenopausal osteoporosis and vertebral fractures. Oestrogen decreased bone turnover with lower levels of osteocalcin and improved BMD at the lumbar spine, femoral trochanter and mid-radius but not the femoral neck. Fewer new fractures were experienced by the oestrogen group (8 fractures in 7 women) compared to the placebo group (20 fractures in 12 women).

A larger study compared HRT, vitamin D, HRT + vitamin D and placebo in 464 non-osteoporotic women. There was a significant reduction in non-vertebral fractures in the HRT group.

Table 6.5 Minimum doses of oestrogen required for osteoporosis prevention	
Method of administration	Dose
Orally	0.3–0.625 mg conjugated oestrogens daily 1–2 mg oestradiol daily 1.25 mg oestrone daily
Transdermally	50 mg oestradiol daily
Subcutaneously	25–100 mg oestradiol 4–6 monthly depending on hormone levels

The recently published Women's Health Initiative, the first large randomized controlled trial of HRT in healthy women, showed a reduced risk of fracture within the HRT group (RR 0.66).

Recent studies have shown that low doses of HRT are effective in improving bone density in older women (>65 years of age). Older women are also more likely to experience side-effects with standard doses of HRT and opting for a lower dose may be more appropriate (Table 6.5).

Duration of HRT use

If BMD were the only consideration and there were no increased risks with long-term use of HRT, then maximum benefit would be obtained if HRT were used lifelong after the menopause. Cohort studies have shown that current and recent users have the lowest risk of osteoporotic fractures. There is also evidence that bone loss increases after HRT is stopped.

A pragmatic length of HRT use is considered to be 7-10 years after menopause at an average age of 50 years to minimize the increased risk of breast cancer associated with long-term use (see Chapter 9). This time limit should not apply to women who have undergone a premature menopause and where HRT use before the age of 50 is replacing 'normal' hormones.

Women should be encouraged to use HRT for 7–10 years after average age of menopause to contribute to osteoporosis prevention.

The issue of limiting long-term use of HRT is more complex if the woman is experiencing menopausal symptoms and wishes to continue with HRT to improve her quality of life. There are other effective options available for the management of osteoporosis (see below) but those for the management of menopausal symptoms are limited.

HRT and other risk factors

A number of studies have shown that the effects of HRT interact with other risk factors. In one, smokers were shown to have half the serum level of oestradiol compared with non-smokers for a given dose of HRT (1 or 2 mg oestradiol) and a low body mass index (BMI) was associated with a higher rate of bone loss in the perimenopause. Unlike smoking, a low BMI responded well to both 1 and 2 mg of oestradiol.

A large retrospective study of 6159 postmenopausal women showed that the protective effect of HRT was more pronounced in certain groups. Although smokers appear to have lower oestradiol levels for a given dose of HRT, the protective effects of HRT were strongest among:

- smokers
- alcohol drinkers
- women who had a sedentary lifestyle.

Tibolone

Tibolone is a synthetic steroid with weak oestrogenic, progestrogenic and androgenic effects. It is effective at treating menopausal symptoms and several studies have shown a significant improvement in BMD when compared with placebo. It has minimal effect on the endometrium and may also improve libido.

Progestogens

Progestogens have a positive effect on bone mass, albeit much weaker than oestrogen. For women who have contraindications to the use of oestrogen and for those who opt not to take HRT, some progestogens (particularly norethisterone), as well as having a positive effect on menopausal symptoms, may be useful in preventing bone loss.

Selective oestrogen receptor modulators (SERMs)

Although tamoxifen has a positive effect on bone, it also stimulates the endometrium, leading to increased rates of vaginal bleeding and endometrial cancers.

Raloxifene is the first SERM to be developed specifically to treat osteoporosis. In a large randomized controlled trial in 7705 osteoporotic women, BMD was significantly higher and the relative risk of vertebral fractures was 0.5–0.7 in the raloxifene-treated group. It had little effect on the endometrium with similar rates of vaginal bleeding in the placebo and raloxifene groups. The raloxifene group also appeared to have a much lower incidence of breast cancer, which is potentially a very important finding. Unfortunately, raloxifene is not useful in the management of menopausal symptoms and, as with oestrogen, it causes a two- to three-fold increase in the incidence of venous thromboembolic disease. It may be most suitable for postmenopausal women without vasomotor symptoms, as even a small increase in breast carcinoma risk associated with long-term conventional HRT can be unacceptable to the asymptomatic woman.

Bisphosphonates

This class of drug inhibits the activity of osteoclasts, resulting in a decrease in bone resorption. These non-hormonal preparations significantly improve BMD and reduce fracture rates for postmenopausal women. There is, however, some need for caution regarding their long-term effects as they have only been widely used for about 10 years.

Biphosphonates significantly reduce fracture rates in postmenopausal women

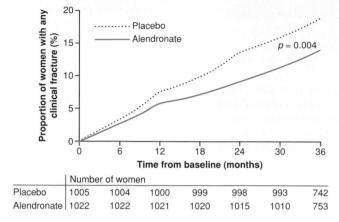

	Number of women						
Placebo	1005	1004	1000	999	998	993	742
Alendronate	1022	1022	1021	1020	1015	1010	753

Figure 6.7
Cumulative proportion of women treated with alendronate or placebo with any clinical fracture. (Reproduced with permission from Elsevier Science; Black DM, Cummings SR, Karpf DB *et al.* Randomised trial of effect of alendronate on risk of fracture in women with existing vertebral fractures. *Lancet* 1996: 348: 1535-41.)

Bisphosphonates are poorly absorbed orally and there have been reports of oesophageal ulceration in some patients. They should be avoided in patients with peptic ulcer disease. It is recommended that biphosphonates are taken with at least 100 ml of water and that the patient remains upright for at least 30 min after ingestion. This can be inconvenient for some patients and biphosphonates are unsuitable for patients who have difficulty understanding administration instructions – a new weekly dosing regime of 70 mg of alendronate is more convenient.

High continuous doses of etidronate are associated with impaired mineralization. However, cyclical etidronate (400 mg daily for 14 days followed by 500 mg calcium daily for 76 days) has been shown to improve bone density significantly and reduce the rate of vertebral fracture by 50% in postmenopausal osteoporosis.

The effects of alendronate on postmenopausal osteoporosis have been extensively studied by the Fracture Intervention Trial Research Group. Women with a low femoral-neck density and at least one existing vertebral fracture were randomized to either placebo or alendronate

(initially 5 mg, later increased to 10 mg). A 3-year follow-up period demonstrated a reduced rate of radiographic and clinical vertebral and non-vertebral fractures in the alendronate group (Figure 6.7).

The Fracture Intervention Trial Research Group later published the results for women with a low femoral neck BMD but no vertebral fracture. In a 4-year follow-up BMD was increased in all sites studied; clinical fractures were reduced, but not significantly so, as was the incidence of radiographically diagnosed vertebral fractures. Subgroup analysis showed a 56% reduction in risk of hip fracture in women with a femoral neck T score of –2.5 or less, but no significant effect in those who had a femoral T score greater than –2.5.

Several large randomized controlled trials have shown that risedronate is effective in reducing both vertebral and non-vertebral fractures in women with osteoporosis. The largest study (n=9300) demonstrated a:

- 39% reduction in risk of hip fracture in women with a low femoral BMD
- 56% reduction in risk in those with a low BMD and a previous vertebral fracture.

Bisphosphonates and oestrogen may have synergistic effects. In a study of 425 hysterectomized women with a low bone mass, BMD was highest when alendronate was added to conjugated oestrogen (8.3% increase in spinal BMD) compared to alendronate alone (increase of 6.0%), oestrogen alone (increase of 6.0%) or placebo (decrease of 0.6%). Bisphosphonates have also been licensed for prevention of osteoporosis in those with risk factors.

Calcitonin

Calcitonin is a polypeptide hormone produced by the C cells of the thyroid gland. It binds to osteoclasts and inhibits bone resorption. It is available as an intramuscular injection or nasal spray. Calcitonin has been shown to improve bone density; however, there is no evidence for a reduction in fracture rates. It is expensive and its use is mainly limited to the acute management of vertebral fractures as it has an analgesic effect.

Further reading

Black DM, Cummings SR, Karpf DB et al. Randomised trial of effect of alendronate on risk of fracture in women with existing vertebral fractures. Lancet 1996; 348: 1531–41.

Chapuy MC, Arlot ME, Duboeuf F et al. Vitamin D and calcium to prevent hip fractures in elderly women. N Engl J Med 1992; 327: 1637–42.

Chevalley T, Rizzoli R, Nydegger V et al. Effects of calcium supplements on femoral bone density and vertebral fracture rate in vitamin D replete elderly patients. Osteoporosis Int 1994; 4: 245–52.

Compston JE, Cooper C, Kanis JA. Fortnightly review: bone densitometry in clinical practice. Br Med J 1995; 310: 1507–10.

Cumming SR, Browner WS, Bauer D et al. Endogenous hormone and the risk of hip and vertebral fractures among older women. Study of osteoporotic fractures research group. N Engl J Med 1998; 339: 733–8.

Ettinger B, Black DM, Mitlak BH et al. Reduction of vertebral fracture risk in postmenopausal women with osteoporosis treated with raloxifene: results from a 3 year randomised clinical trial. JAMA 1999; 282: 637–45.

Gotfredson A, Nilas L, Riis BJ et al. Bone changes occurring spontaneously and caused by ostrogen in early postmenopausal women: a local or generalised phenomenon. Br Med J Clin Res Edition 1986; 292: 1098–100.

Harris ST, Watts NB, Genant HK et al. Effects of risedronate treatment on vertebral and non-vertebral fractures in women with postmenopausal osteoporosis: a randomised controlled trial. Vertebral Efficacy With Risedronate Therapy (VERT) Study Group. JAMA 1999; 282: 1344–52.

Hoidrup S, Gronbaek M, Pedersen AT et al. Hormone replacement therapy and hip fracture risk: effect modification by tobacco smoking, alcohol intake, physical activity, and body mass index. Am J Epidemiol 1999; 150: 1085–93.

Horowitz M, Wishart JM, Need AG et al. Effects of norethisterone on bone related biochemical variables and forearm bone density in postmenopausal osteoporosis. Clin Endocrinol 1993; 39: 649–55.

Kiel DP, Felson DT, Anderson JJ et al. Hip fracture and the use of estrogens in postmenopausal women, The Framingham Study. N Engl J Med 1987; 317: 1169–74.

Komulainen MH, Kroger H, Tuppurainen MT et al. HRT and Vit D in the prevention of non-vertebral fractures in postmenopausal women; a 5 year randomised trial. Maturitas 1998; 31: 45–54.

Lindsay R, Hart DM, Forrest C et al. Prevention of spinal osteoporosis in oophoorectomised women. Lancet 1980; 2: 1151–4.

Lufkin EG, Wahner HW, O'Fallon WM et al. Treatment of postmenopausal osteoporosis with transdermal oestrogen. Ann Intern Med 1992; 117: 1–9.

Marshall D, Johnell O, Wedel H. Meta-analysis of how well measures of bone mineral density predict occurrence of osteoporotic fractures. Br Med J 1996; 312: 1254–9.

Pols HAP, Felsenberg D, Hanley DA et al. Multinational, placebo-controlled, randomised trial of the effects of alendronate on bone density and fracture risk in postmenopausal women with low bone mass, results of the FOSIT study. Osteoporosis Int 1999; 9: 461–8.

Recker RR, Davies M, Dowd RM et al. The effect of low-dose continuous estrogen and progesterone with calcium and vitamin D on bone in elderly women: randomised, controlled trial. Ann Int Med 1999; 130: 897–904.

Reginster JY, Denis D, Deroisy R et al. Longterm (3 years) prevention of trabecular postmenopausal bone loss with low-dose intermittent nasal calcitonin. J Bone Min Res 1994; 9: 69–73.

Reginster JY, Minne HW, Sorensen OH et al. Randomised trial of the effects of risedronate on vertebral fractures in women with established postmenopausal osteoporosis. Osteoporosis Int 2000; 11: 83–91.

Rymer J, Chapman MG, Foghelman I. Effect of tibolone on postmenopausal bone loss. Osteoporosis Int 1994; 4: 314–19.

Torgerson DJ, Dolan P. Prescribing by general practitioners after an osteoporotic fracture. Ann Rheum Dis 1998; 7: 378–9.

Watts NB, Harsi ST, Genant HK. Intermittent cyclical etidronate treatment of postmenopausal osteoporosis. N Engl J Med 1990; 323: 73–9.

Writing group for the Women's Health Initiative. Risks and benefits of estrogen plus progestin in healthy postmenopausal women. JAMA 2002; 288: 321–33.

7. Hormone replacement therapy and arterial disease

Protective effect of HRT use
Increase in cardiovascular risk
  with HRT use in prospective
  randomized trials
HRT and blood pressure
Current recommendations
Prescribing for women at high risk of
  coronary heart disease

Protective effect of HRT use

There is a wealth of observational and epidemiological data suggesting that women who choose to take HRT have a significantly lower risk of coronary heart disease (CHD). Meta-analyses of such studies have calculated a pooled relative risk of CHD of 0.64 (95% CI 0.59–0.68) for ever-users versus never-users of HRT and 0.5 (95% CI 0.45–0.59) for current users of oestrogen versus non-users. Also, data from the large prospective Nurses study, involving 59,337 women followed for 16 years, found an adjusted relative risk of CHD of 0.6 (95% CI 0.43–0.83) for oestrogen users versus never-users.

> HRT appeared to significantly reduce the risk of coronary heart disease

However, epidemiological studies may demonstrate a degree of selection bias, in that women who choose to take HRT may have a healthier lifestyle with fewer environmental risk behaviours than women who do not. In addition, the consistency in the gradient of the CHD incidence curve at the time of the menopause confounds the proposed importance of oestrogen deficiency.

Increase in cardiovascular risk with HRT use in prospective randomized trials

In light of the largely positive observational trial data concerning HRT and CHD risk reduction, a randomized placebo-controlled trial, The Heart and Estrogen/Progestin Replacement Study (HERS), was undertaken to study the effect of daily conjugated equine estrogens (CEE) plus medroxyprogesterone acetate (MPA) on the combined rate of nonfatal myocardial infarction (MI) and CHD-related deaths among postmenopausal women with established coronary disease. The mean age of the participants was 67 years and more than 55% had a body mass index of >27 kg/m^2. The results were surprising and have had a significant effect on the use of HRT for CHD risk reduction. Overall, there was no difference in event rates in the hormone (172 events or CHD deaths) and placebo groups (176 events or CHD deaths), with a relative hazard (RH) of 0.99 (95% CI 0.80–1.22) over a mean follow-up of 4.1 years. However, there was a significant time trend with a greater number of CHD events observed in the first year of use in women randomized to take HRT as compared with placebo [RH 1.52 (95% CI 1.01–1.29)] compared with years 4 and 5 [RH 0.67 (95% CI0.43–1.04)].

> HRT may actually increase the risk of coronary events in the first year of use

The researchers correctly cautioned against commencing HRT in women with CHD, for the purpose of secondary prevention of acute events. However, given the favourable trend of CHD events after several years of therapy, they suggested that women with CHD who are established on HRT could be advised to continue with it (as depicted in line B in Figure 7.1).

The recent report from the Women's Health Initiative (WHI) study, a placebo-controlled primary prevention trial of oral oestrogen (CEE)

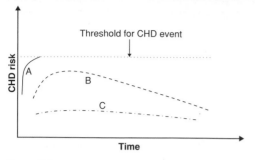

Figure 7.1

Postulated patterns of change in coronary heart disease (CHD) risk over time with differing HRT regimens. A, This line represents an early increase in CHD risk, potentially mediated by procoagulant, proinflammatory effects of oral oestrogens and increased triglyceride concentrations, sufficient to provoke a CHD event in some women taking HRT; B, in this case, the early increase in CHD risk is insufficient to provoke a CHD event and in subsequent years CHD risk lessens due in part to favourable effects of oral oestrogens on low-density lipoprotein (LDL) and high-density lipoprotein (HDL) cholesterol concentrations, although other effects of oral oestrogens are likely to come into play; C, this line illustrates the potential early and late impact of transdermal oestrogens, which by avoidance of hepatic first-pass metabolism may lessen any early increase in CHD risk due to smaller effects on proinflammatory, procoagulant and triglyceride pathways. However, later beneficial effects may be minimized with transdermal oestrogens as HDL- and LDL-cholesterol effects are also reduced.

plus progestogen (MPA) (ie the same preparation as used in HERS) in younger healthy postmenopausal women, also reported an excess of cardiovascular events in the HRT group. Indeed, for every 10,000 person-years attributable to CEE combined with MPA there were seven more CHD events and eight more strokes. The authors therefore recommed that this regimen should not be initiated or continued for primary prevention of CHD.

How far HERS and WHI results can be extrapolated is uncertain since the HRT used in these studies was untypical of preparations used in the UK where oestradiol-based preparations are more common. The progestogen MPA is also less commonly used in the UK compared to the USA.

Proposed explanations for early excess risk

Several mechanisms have been implicated, including inflammation and coagulation. Additionally, elevations in serum triglyceride concentration must be considered. The nature of the oestrogen and progestogen, and the dose and route of delivery, may also be implicated in determining early changes in CHD risk.

Table 7.1 shows the relative changes occurring in a range of risk factors with different hormonal preparations.

Lipids

Oral oestrogens increase cardioprotective HDL-cholesterol and decrease LDL-cholesterol. Such lipid effects appear greater with oral conjugated equine oestrogen (CEE) than oestradiol and are negligible with transdermal delivery of oestradiol due to avoidance of hepatic first-pass metabolism.

On the negative side, oral oestrogens also increase circulating triglyceride concentrations and, once again, such effects are more pronounced with CEE than oestradiol and are negligible with transdermal preparations. Triglyceride is an independent risk factor for CHD, particularly in women; raised concentrations can promote adverse effects on:

- platelets
- endothelium
- coagulation
- vascular inflammation.

All of these effects are linked to greater arterial plaque instability. It has been calculated that even after correcting for other risk factors, including HDL-cholesterol, the relative risk of CHD increases by 37% in women for each 1 mmol/l increase in plasma triglyceride concentration. Therefore, although both LDL- and HDL-cholesterol concentrations improved with HRT use in the HERS study (11% decrease and 10% increase, respectively), it can be speculated that the

Table 7.1
Metabolic changes with different HRT preparations and routes of administration

	Oestrogen component				Progesterone component	
	Oral CEE	Oral E$_2$ (2 mg)	Oral E$_2$ (1 mg)	E$_2$ (transdermal)	Oral MPA	Oral norethisterone
Lipids:						
Triglyceride	↑↑	↑	↑/→	→	↓	↓
HDL-cholesterol	↑↑	↑↑	↑	→	↓	↓
LDL-cholesterol	↓↓	↓↓	↓	→	→	→
Coagulation:						
Factor VII		↑↑	↑↑	↑	↓	↓
C-reactive protein	↑↑	↑	→	ND/→	ND	↓

CEE = conjugated equine oestrogen; E$_2$ = oestradiol; MPA = medroxyprogesterone acetate; ND = not done.

10% increase in triglyceride could have contributed to an early increase in CHD events by promoting greater plaque instability. However, in later years, the LDL- and HDL-cholesterol changes may have stabilized the progression of atherosclerosis so that CHD risk subsequently decreased.

Progestogens oppose the oestrogen-induced elevations in HDL-cholesterol and triglyceride concentrations in proportion to the degree of androgenicity. Since most of the focus has been to try to maintain the beneficial HDL-cholesterol effects, most observers have advocated the addition of less androgenic progestogens into combined HRT preparations. As a result, MPA was the chosen progestogen in HERS rather than a more androgenic progestogen such as norethisterone, which is known to attenuate or even reverse the HDL- and triglyceride-raising effects of oestrogens.

Coagulation and fibrinolysis

Short-term oral oestrogen alone, or in combination with progestogen, shifts the procoagulant-anticoagulant balance towards a procoagulant state. Oral oestrogen is associated with a rise in clotting factors, such as Factor VII, and markers of thrombin generation (prothrombin fragments F$_{1+2}$ and fibrinopeptide A). A significant reduction in

fibrinogen has also been observed. The naturally occurring anticoagulants antithrombin and protein S fall in a dose-dependent manner in association with oral oestrogen.

Fibrinolysis is another important aspect of haemostasis that appears to be altered by HRT. A number of studies suggest an increase in fibrinolysis and reduction in plasminogen activator inhibitor-1 (PAI-1) in association with the administration of oral oestrogen or combined oral oestrogen and progestogen.

These findings were not reproduced when oestradiol was administered transdermally. A reduction in tissue plasminogen activator (tPA) in association with oral oestrogens may impair fibrinolysis and, therefore, enhance this adverse procoagulant shift. The liver is an important organ in the manufacture and metabolism of coagulation factors; avoiding first-pass metabolism, as occurs with transdermal HRT, may reduce some of the hormone effects on the production and metabolism of haemostatic variables. These data are consistent with the suggestion of lower deep venous thrombosis (DVT) rates with transdermal HRT preparations (see Chapter 8).

Studies in which transdermal oestradiol has been combined with oral MPA or norethisterone have shown significant reductions in Factor VII activity. However, comprehensive data on other effects of progestogens on coagulation and fibrinolysis pathways are generally lacking with regards to HRT.

Inflammation

C-reactive protein (CRP) is a marker of inflammation and strongly predicts the occurrence of cardiovascular events in healthy men and women. In a recent prospective case-control study in postmenopausal women, the only risk markers independently to predict CHD risk were CRP and total cholesterol:HDL-cholesterol ratio. It is significant, therefore, that three recent studies have reported an approximately two-fold increase in CRP with oral HRT in postmenopausal women, raising the possibility that the increased risk of cardiovascular events after starting HRT is related to an initial increase in CRP levels. An increase in CRP may reflect an overall net proinflammatory action of HRT, thereby increasing plaque instability. Alternatively, because CRP localizes in infarcted myocardium (with colocalization of activated complement), it is possible that CRP may directly interact with atherosclerotic vessels or ischaemic myocardium by activation of the complement system, thereby promoting local inflammation and thrombosis. It should be noted, however, that oral oestrogens reduce IL-6 levels, a major promoter of hepatic CRP synthesis, so that the inflammation picture is by no means simple.

In a small study of 27 women, 1 mg of oestradiol daily sequentially combined with dydrogesterone did not increase CRP levels, but 2 mg oestradiol increased levels significantly, raising the possibility that the CRP increase is dose-dependent.

There are no data concerning the effects of transdermal oestrogen alone. However, there is evidence that caeruloplasmin, a positive acute phase reactant, increases with oral oestrogen replacement but not transdermal oestrogen

replacement. Furthermore, in a double-blind, placebo-controlled trial in women with type 2 diabetes, a reduction in CRP concentration was seen with a combination of transdermal oestradiol and continuous oral norethisterone. This suggests that androgenic progestogens may reduce CRP concentrations, an observation in keeping with the previously noted anti-inflammatory effects of both progestogens and androgens.

It seems that elevations in CRP may be minimized at lower doses of oestradiol (1 mg) or by use of transdermal oestrogens, and attenuated or reversed with the addition of oral androgenic progestogens.

HRT and blood pressure

Although blood pressure can increase with the oral contraceptive, most trials with HRT show no increase in either systolic or diastolic blood pressure. Some trials even suggest a potential fall in blood pressure with HRT and a reduced blood pressure variability. However, these trials have often been inadequately controlled and powered.

A randomized double-blind study of oestradiol combined with a progestogen demonstrated no increase in blood pressure, providing some reassurance that HRT need not be withheld in hypertensive women. It is suggested that blood pressure is checked prior to and at least once shortly after starting a woman on HRT. There is probably no need to check blood pressure more frequently than indicated on clinical grounds unless the HRT regimen is altered.

> HRT does not appear to increase blood pressure

Current recommendations

As a consequence of HERS and WHI, it is recommended that HRT should not be started for cardioprotection in women with existing CHD. Women with CHD who are already on HRT are now advised to consult their doctor to discuss the possible benefits and risks of HRT.

If a woman is at high risk of CHD, as judged by a comprehensive assessment of major risk factors, then it would seem prudent to use medication of proven value for CHD risk reduction, eg aspirin or statin therapy (if indicated by reputable CHD risk charts), rather than HRT. It is suggested that HRT should only be prescribed for indications such as relief of menopausal symptoms and osteoporosis prophylaxis.

Prescribing for women at high risk of CHD

Many women who would benefit from HRT for menopausal symptoms or osteoporosis prophylaxis have an elevated risk of CHD. From available data, it may be possible to predict those HRT preparations which provide a more favourable physiological response and, therefore, are more suitable for such women. Preparations that contain low-dose oestradiol rather than CEE, and that are transdermally rather than orally administered, may be more suitable as they have potentially less effect on pathways implicated in increasing plaque instability, and consequently avoid the potential early increase in CHD risk seen with oral CEE-based preparations. The North American Menopause Society reached broadly similar conclusions in a recent consensus statement for women with type 2 diabetes. The recent WHI results may widen the use of lower-dose HRT for all women, regardless of their CHD risk status.

> Women with an increased risk of CHD requiring HRT for symptoms or bone protection should be prescribed transdermal, or low-dose oral oestradiol HRT preparations

The ideal choice of progestogen remains unclear, but androgenic progestogens should not necessarily be overlooked and may have particular advantages. Moreover, MPA appears to have some adverse metabolic effects and can worsen insulin sensitivity. Norethisterone appears to be neutral with respect to insulin sensitivity.

Further reading

Barrett-Connor E, Grady D. Hormone replacement therapy, heart disease, and other considerations. *Annu Rev Pub Health* 1998; **19**: 55–72.

Castellsague J, Pereez Guttann S *et al*. Recent epidemiological studies of the association between hormone replacement therapy and venous thromboembolism. A review. *Drug Safety* 1998; **18**: 117–23.

Cushman M, Legault C, Barrett-Connor E *et al*. Effect of postmenopausal hormones on inflammation-sensitive proteins: the Postmenopausal Estrogen/Progestin Interventions (PEPI) Study. *Circulation* 1999; **100**: 717–22.

Grodstein F, Stampfer MJ, Manson JE *et al*. Postmenopausal estrogen and progestin use and the risk of cardiovascular disease. *N Engl J Med* 1996; **335**: 453–61. [Published erratum in *N Engl J Med* 1996; **335**: 1406.]

Hulley S, Grady D, Bush T *et al*. Randomized trial of estrogen plus progestin for secondary prevention of coronary heart disease in postmenopausal women. Heart and Estrogen/progestin Replacement Study (HERS) Research Group. *JAMA* 1998; **280**: 605–13.

Kornhauser C, Malacara JM, Garay ME, Perez-Luque EL. The effect of hormone replacement therapy on blood pressure and cardiovascular risk factors in menopausal women with moderate hypertension. *J Hum Hypertens* 1997; **11**: 405–11.

Kroon UB, Silfverstolpe G, Tengborn L. The effects of transdermal estradiol and oral conjugated estrogens on haemostasis variables. *Thromb Haemostas* 1994; **71**: 420–3.

Larkin M. Ups and downs for HRT and heart disease. *Lancet* 2000; **355**: 1338.

Ridker PM, Hennekens CH, Buring JE, Rifai N. C-reactive protein and other markers of inflammation in the prediction of cardiovascular disease in women. *N Engl J Med* 2000; **342**: 836–43.

Sattar N, Perera M, Small M, Lumsden MA. Hormone replacement therapy and sensitive C-reactive protein concentrations in women with type-2 diabetes. *Lancet* 1999; **354**: 487–8.

The North American Menopause Society. Effects of menopause and oestrogen replacement therapy or hormone replacement therapy in women with diabetes mellitus: consensus opinion of The North American Menopause Society. *Menopause* 2000; **7**: 87–95.

The Writing Group for the PEPI Trial. Effects of estrogen or estrogen/progestin regimens on heart disease risk factors in post-menopausal women. The postmenopausal Estrogen/Progestin Interventions trial. *JAMA* 1995; **273**: 199–208.

Van Baal WM, Emeis JJ, van der Mooren MJ *et al*. Impaired procoagulant-anticoagulant balance during hormone replacement therapy? A randomised placebo-controlled 12-week study. *Thromb Haemostas* 2000; **83**: 29–34.

Van Baal WM, Kenemans P, van der Mooren MJ *et al.* Increased C-reactive protein levels during short-term hormone replacement therapy in healthy postmenopausal women. *Thromb Haemostas* 1999; **81**: 925–8.

Writing group for the Women's Health Initiative. Risks and benefits of estrogen plus progestin in healthy postmenopausal women. *JAMA* 2002; **288**: 321–33.

8. Hormone replacement therapy and venous thromboembolism

HRT-associated risk of venous thromboembolism
Relative risk of HRT
Recommendations for management

HRT-associated risk of venous thromboembolism

Hormone replacement therapy (HRT) was not, until recently, considered to be a risk factor for venous thromboembolism (VTE), but many of the initial studies assessing the risk had limited statistical power or methodological limitations. More recent case-control studies have shown an increase in the relative risk of VTE in women using oestrogen-containing HRT (Table 8.1).

> HRT increases the relative risk of venous thromboembolism

These studies consistently show an increased relative risk of VTE, although the absolute risk, in the absence of other risk factors, is low. The exception is the HERS study, which showed a much higher absolute risk of VTE. However, the population studied was at much greater risk of VTE because of coexisting medical conditions associated with both heart disease and VTE. The dose of oestrogen may also be a factor as two studies reported that the relative risk of VTE increased as the dose of oestrogen increased. Transdermal oestrogen replacement therapy may carry a lower risk of VTE although data on these preparations are very limited.

Table 8.1
Risk of thrombosis and thromboembolism with hormone replacement therapy

Type of study	Relative risk
Population-based case-control study	3.6 (95% CI 1.6–7.8), dependent on oestrogen dose, for current users for idiopathic VTE. (Absolute risk per 100,000 women per year – 32 for users compared with 9 for non-users)
Hospital-based case-control study	3.5 (95% CI 1.8–7.0) for idiopathic VTE in current HRT users aged 45–64 years. Highest risk among short-term current users. (Absolute risk per 100,000 women per year – 27 for users compared with 11 for non-users)
Questionnaire study on Nurses Health Cohort	2.1 (95% CI 1.2–3.8) for idiopathic primary PTE in current HRT users
Population-based case-control study	2.1 (95% CI 1.4–3.2) for current HRT users for idiopathic VTE. Increase in risk restricted to first year of use
Case-control study	2.3 (95% CI 1.0–5.3) for current HRT users for idiopathic VTE. Increase in risk restricted to first year of use
Randomized, double-blind, placebo-controlled trial of HRT for secondary prevention of coronary heart disease (HERS)	VTE: 2.7 (95% CI 1.4–5.0), DVT: 2.8 (95% CI 1.3–6.0), PTE: 2.8 (95% CI 0.9–8.7) for current HRT users. Absolute risk for VTE per 100,000 women per year – 620 for users compared with 230 for non-users
Randomized, double-blind, placebo-controlled trial of HRT for the primary prevention of coronary heart disease (WHI)	VTE: 2.11 (95% CI 1.26–3.55), DVT: 2.07 (95% CI 1.14–3.74), PTE: 2.13 (95% CI 0.99–4.56)
Population-based case-control study	3.54 (95% CI 1.54–8.2) in first 12 months of oestradiol-containing HRT use for VTE, reducing thereafter to 0.66 (95% CI 0.39–1.11)

PTE, pulmonary thromboembolism; VTE, venous thromboembolism; DVT, deep venous thrombosis

The frequency of VTE in postmenopausal women is around twice that of premenopausal women. However, as the risk of VTE is higher in the first year of HRT exposure, the interaction of age and HRT cannot be responsible for the increased risk of VTE.

Possible mechanisms

There are several potential mechanisms underlying the link between HRT and VTE.

Coagulation, fibrinolysis and inflammation

Several changes in the coagulation and fibrinolytic systems occur naturally after the menopause, ie increasing levels of:

- Factor VII
- Factor VIII
- fibrinogen
- the body's endogenous anticoagulants
- antithrombin
- protein C.

Oral HRT is associated with a reduction in plasma levels of fibrinogen, Factor VII, von Willebrand Factor and antithrombin. Conversely, fibrinolysis is enhanced. It is also known to provoke an increase in resistance to activated protein C. This is of interest as there is an established association between resistance to activated protein C and venous thrombosis, independent of HRT. These effects on the coagulation system are associated with increased thrombin generation, indicating activation of the coagulation system. Some of the effects of HRT on coagulation and fibrinolysis therefore appear beneficial, while others appear detrimental with regard to risk of VTE.

Proinflammatory changes in the body are also recognized as a risk factor for VTE. C-reactive protein (CRP, an inflammatory marker produced by the liver) levels in the blood are increased with oestrogen-containing HRT.

Transdermal oestrogen preparations, which avoid the first-pass effect in the liver, have a lesser effect on coagulation factors produced by the liver than oral HRT. A large study has reported that oral, but not transdermal, HRT is associated with increased plasma levels of Factor IX, activated protein C resistance and CRP, and reduced levels of tissue plasminogen activator and plasminogen activator inhibitor.

Thrombophilic phenotype

One possibility is that HRT might precipitate a venous thrombosis in women with inherited or acquired thrombophilia. Heritable thrombophilias have a prevalence of 15–20% in Western European populations. Clearly, the incidence of VTE is much lower than this and it is now established that additional risk factors are usually required before a clinical VTE will occur in people with an inherited thrombophilia. Hyperhomocysteineaemia is a risk factor for venous thrombosis. It is frequently the result of a combination of genotype [homozygotes for the so-called thermolabile (C677T) variant of methylene tetrohydrofolate reductase (10% prevalence) are at risk] and an acquired dietary deficiency in B vitamins, such as folic acid. However, as HRT reduces serum homocysteine, this is unlikely to account for the excess risk of VTE with HRT.

> It is possible that HRT may cause a venous thrombosis in females with inherited or acquired thrombophilia

A case-control study has assessed whether a thrombophilic phenotype is associated with an increased risk of VTE when combined with HRT. VTE was significantly associated with HRT use, activated protein C resistance, low antithrombin and high Factor IX. Irrespective of the underlying prothrombotic tendency, HRT resulted in around a three-fold increase in the risk of VTE. There is a substantial increase in risk of VTE when multiple risk factors are present; the estimated odds ratio for VTE is over 150 for a woman on HRT with increased Factor IX, activated protein C resistance and low antithrombin. Thus, multiple acquired and/or inherited risk factors for VTE, including HRT, are necessary for a clinical thrombosis to occur.

Relative risk of HRT

It would appear that HRT should now be added to the list of established risk factors for VTE, which include:

- thrombophilia
- age
- obesity
- varicose veins
- previous VTE
- deep venous insufficiency
- immobility
- trauma or surgery
- malignancy
- cardiac failure
- paralysis of lower limbs
- infection
- inflammatory bowel disease
- nephrotic syndrome.

One case-control study has put this risk in context by assessing the relative risk of various risk factors for VTE; obesity and varicose veins carried a greater risk than HRT (Table 8.2). However, it should be noted that there is potential for significant interaction between risk factors. A randomized double-blind placebo-controlled trial of HRT (2 mg estradiol plus 1 mg norethisterone) in 140 women with a previous VTE found that the incidence of VTE was 10.7% in the HRT group and 2.3% in the placebo group within 262 days of starting therapy. There was no difference between these groups in terms of additional risk factors, including thrombophilia.

Recommendations for management

These are summarized in Table 8.3.

There is no indication to screen for thrombophilia prior to starting or continuing HRT in the woman with no personal history of VTE and no family history of thrombophilia. However, when a woman starts or continues HRT it is important to assess for the presence of other risk factors for venous thrombosis, and

Table 8.2
Association of VTE and risk factors including HRT

Risk factor	Adjusted odds ratio (95% CI)
Varicose veins	6.9 (4.3–11.0)
Obesity	4.6 (2.2–9.7)
Osteoarthritis	2.4 (1.7–3.3)
Age (65–80 vs 45–64 years)	2.3 (1.6–3.2)
HRT (current use)	1.9 (1.2–2.3)
Hypertension	1.6 (1.2–2.3)

[From: Varas-Lorenzo C, Gracia-Rodriguez LA, Cattaruzzi C et al. Hormone replacement therapy and the risk of hospitalization for venous thromboembolism: A population-based study. Am J Epidemiol 1998; **147**: 387–90.]

specifically for a personal history of DVT or PTE, or a history of VTE in a first- or second-degree relative. Screening for thrombophilia should be offered if a woman has such a personal or family history of VTE. In addition, in women over 50 years of age with a recent VTE, the possibility of underlying malignancy or connective tissue disease should be considered.

Table 8.3
Recommendations for minimization of risk of VTE in women taking HRT

- There is no indication to perform universal screening for thrombophilia prior to starting or continuing HRT
- Assess for the presence of other risk factors for venous thrombosis prior to starting or continuing HRT
- Offer screening for thrombophilia if a woman has a personal or family history of VTE
- Avoid HRT if possible if a woman has multiple risk factors for VTE
- Avoid oral HRT if a woman has had a previous VTE, regardless of whether she has a known thrombophilia
- Refer women with thrombophilia and no previous VTE to a clinician with special expertise in thrombophilia
- Do not routinely stop HRT prior to surgery. If thromboprophylaxis with low-dose or low molecular weight heparin with or without thromboembolic deterrent stockings are used, HRT can be continued

> A woman starting HRT should be assessed for the presence of risk factors for venous thrombosis

If a woman has multiple risk factors for VTE, HRT, which is an additional risk factor, should probably be avoided, but the woman's overall situation should be taken into account. Where the woman has had a previous VTE, regardless of whether she has a known thrombophilia, oral HRT should usually be avoided because of the relatively high risk of recurrent thrombosis. If HRT is considered necessary for such a patient, transdermal therapy may be best as it has less effect on the coagulation system than oral HRT. The woman must also be counselled about the risk of recurrent VTE. Strategies, such as anticoagulant 'cover', can be considered for the period during which HRT is required, but the risk of haemorrhagic complications from the anticoagulant therapy must be taken into account in assessing the usefulness of this strategy. Women on long-term anticoagulation because of a thrombotic problem need not avoid HRT, but transdermal therapy may be best. These situations pose difficult management decisions and merit specialist advice from clinicians with expertise in the management of thrombophilia and venous thrombosis.

Women with no personal history of VTE, but who have a thrombophilia identified through screening because of a family history of VTE, require individual assessment. HRT should be avoided with thrombophilic problems associated with a high risk of thrombosis, such as antithrombin deficiency and combinations of thrombophilic defects, eg Factor V Leiden homozygotes and Factor V Leiden combined with prothrombin 20210A. For asymptomatic carriers of thrombophilia, such as Factor V Leiden heterozygotes, or prothrombin 20210A heterozygotes with no other risk factors for VTE, HRT can be considered. It is best avoided as these women will have a several-fold increased relative risk of VTE. Again, these women can present difficult management problems and should be referred to a clinician with special expertise in thrombophilia.

HRT has been considered by some clinicians to be a risk factor for postoperative VTE. However, there are no data to support this view. Nonetheless, in view of the association between VTE and HRT, HRT should probably be considered to be a risk factor for postoperative VTE along with other established risk factors, such as obesity, varicose veins and immobility, in the woman's preoperative VTE risk assessment. The risk from HRT alone is likely to be small and virtually all women on HRT will meet the criteria for perioperative thromboprophylaxis as set out in various guidelines. Routinely stopping HRT prior to surgery is not an evidenced-based practice and, provided appropriate thromboprophylaxis such as low-dose or low molecular weight heparin with or without thromboembolic deterrent stockings are used, HRT can be continued.

Further reading

Carter C. Pathogenesis of thrombosis. In: Greer IA, Turpie AGG, Forbes CD, eds. *Haemostasis and Thrombosis in Obstetrics and Gynaecology*. London: Chapman & Hall, 1992: 229–56.

Daly E, Vessey MP, Hawkins MM *et al*. Case control study of venous thromboembolism risk in users of hormone replacement therapy. *Lancet* 1996; **348**: 977–80.

Douketis JD, Gordon M, Johnston M *et al*. The effects of hormone replacement therapy on thrombin generation, fibrinolysis inhibition, and resistance to activated protein C: Prospective cohort and review of the literature. *Thromb Res* 2000; **99**: 25–34.

Grady D, Wenger NK, Herrington D *et al*. Postmenopausal hormone therapy increases risk for venous thromboembolic disease. The heart and estrogen/progestinreplacement study. *Ann Intern Med* 2000; **132**: 689–96.

Grodstein F, Stampfer MJ, Goldhaber SZ *et al*. Prospective study of exogenous hormones and risk of pulmonary embolism in women. *Lancet* 1996; **348**: 983–7.

Gutthann SP, Garcia-Rodrigues LA, Castallsague J, Oliart AD. Hormone replacement therapy and risk of venous thromboembolism: population based case control study. *Br Med J* 1997; **314**: 796–800.

Hoibraaten E, Abdelnoor M, Sandset PM. Hormone replacement therapy with estradiol and risk of venous thromboembolism. *Thromb Haemostas* 1999; **82**: 1218–21.

Hoibraaten E, Qvigstad E, Arnesen H *et al*. Increased risk of recurrent venous thromboembolism during hormone replacement therapy. *Thromb Haemostas* 2000; **84**: 961–67.

Jick H, Derby LE, Myers, MW et al. Risk of hospital admission for idiopathic venous thromboembolism among users of postmenopausal oestrogens. Lancet 1996; **348**: 981–3.

Jick H, Jick SS, Gurewich V et al. Risk of idiopathic cardiovascular death and nonfatal venous thromboembolism in women using oral contraceptives with differing prostagen components. Lancet 1995; **346**: 1589–93.

Koh KK, Mincemoyer R, Bui MN et al. Effects of hormone-replacement therapy on fibrinolysis in postmenopausal women. N Engl J Med 1997; **336**: 683–90.

Greer IA, Walker ID. Hormone replacement therapy and venous thromboembolism. Climacteric 1999; **2**: 1–8.

Lindoff C, Peterson F, Lecander I et al. Transdermal oestrogen replacement therapy: beneficial effects on haemostatic risk factors for cardiovascular disease. Maturitas 1996; **24**: 43–50.

Lip GY, Blann AD, Jones AE, Beevers DG. Effects of hormone replacement therapy on hemostatic factors, lipid factors and endothelial function in women undergoing surgical menopause: implications for prevention of atherosclerosis Am Heart J 1997; **134**: 764–71.

Lowe GD, Greer IA, Cooke TG et al. Thromboembolic Risk Factors (THRIFT) Consensus Group. Risk of and prophylaxis for venous thromboembolism in hospital patients. Br Med J 1992; **305**: 567–74.

Lowe GD, Rumley A, Woodward M et al. Activated protein C resistance and the FV:R506Q mutation in a random population sample: associations with cardiovascular risk factors and coagulation variables. Thromb Haemostas 1999; **81**: 918–24.

Lowe GD, Rumley A, Woodward M et al. Epidemiology of coagulation factors, inhibitors and activation markers: the third Glasgow MONICA Survey 1 illustrative reference ranges by age, sex and hormone use. Br J Haematol 1997; **97**: 775–84.

Lowe GD, Upton MN, Rumley A et al. Different aspects of oral and transdermal hormone replacement therapies on factor IX, APC resistance, t-PA, PAI and C-reactive protein. A cross-sectional population survey. Thromb Haemostas 2001; **86**: 550–6.

Lowe GD, Woodward M, Vessey M et al. Thrombotic variables and risk of idiopathic venous thromboembolism in women aged 45–64 years. Thromb Haemostas 2000; **83**: 530–5.

Meade TW, Dyer S, Howarth DJ et al. Antithrombin III and procoagulant activity: sex differences and effects of the menopause. Br J Haematol 1994; **74**: 77–81.

Nachtigall LE, Nachtigall RH, Nachtigall RD, Beckman EM. Estrogen replacement therapy II. A prospective study in the relationship to carcinoma and cardiovascular and metabolic problems. Obstet Gynecol 1979; **54**: 74–9.

PEPI (The Postmenopausal Estrogen/Progestin Interventions Trial) Writing Group. Effects of estrogen/progestin regimens on heart disease risk factors in postmenopausal women. JAMA 1995; **273**: 199–208.

Pettiti DB, Wingerd J, Pellegrin F, Ramcharan S. Risk of vascular disease in women. JAMA 1979; **242**: 1150–4.

Ridker P, Hennekens C, Rifai N et al. Hormone replacement therapy and increased plasma concentration of C-reactive protein. Circulation 1999; **100**: 713–16.

Rosendaal F. Venous thrombosis: a multicausal disease. Lancet 1999; **353**: 1167–73.

The Writing Group for the Oestradiol Clotting Study. Effects on haemostasis of hormone replacement therapy with transdermal oestradiol and oral sequential medroxyprogesterone acetate: a one year double blind placebo controlled study. Thromb Haemostas 1996; **75**: 476–80.

Van der Mooren MJ, Vouters GAJ, Blom JH et al. Hormone replacement therapy may reduce high serum homocysteine in postmenopausal women. Eur J Clin Invest 1994; **24**: 733–6.

Varas-Lorenzo C, Garcia-Rodriguez LA, Cattaruzzi C et al. Hormone replacement therapy and the risk of hospitalization for venous thromboembolism: A population based study. Am J Epidemiol 1998; **147**: 387–90.

Walker ID. Congenital thrombophilia. In: Greer IA, ed. Thromboembolic disease in obstetrics and gynaecology. Ballieres Clin Obstet Gynaecol 1997; **11**: 431–45.

Whitehead M, Godfree V. Venous thromboembolism and hormone replacement therapy. In: Greer IA, ed. Thromboembolic disease in obstetrics and gynaecology. Ballieres Clin Obstet Gynaecol 1997; **11**: 587–99.

Writing group for the Women's Health Initiative. Risks and benefits of estrogen plus progestin in healthy postmenopausal women. JAMA 2002; **288**: 321–33.

9. Hormone replacement therapy and cancer risk

Endometrial cancer
Breast cancer
Ovarian cancer
Malignant melanoma

Endometrial cancer

Exposure to unopposed oestrogens is a well-proven risk factor for the development of endometrial hyperplasia (Figure 9.1) and potentially for endometrial cancer. This can occur in premenopausal women if they experience long anovulatory episodes, those with polycystic ovarian syndrome being a typical example. Oestrogen-only HRT was used widely in North America until the 1980s and it has been shown that one to five years of unopposed

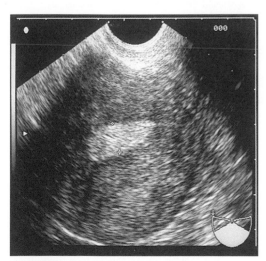

Figure 9.1
Endometrial hyperplasia as imaged by transvaginal ultrasonography. The endometrial thickness is 8.6 mm. (Image courtesy of Dr Linda McMillan, Western Infirmary.)

oestrogens is associated with a three-fold increase in risk of developing endometrial carcinoma when compared to no HRT. With long-term use the risk may be as high as 10-fold.

> Unopposed oestrogens are associated with an increase in the risk of endometrial carcinoma

Role of progesterone

Progesterone inhibits the proliferation and mitosis of the endometrium and the addition of progestogen to HRT preparations significantly reduces the endometrial cancer. In sequential regimes, which mimic the normal menstrual cycle and aim to provide a predictable bleeding pattern, the addition of 13 days of progesterone reduces the risk of endometrial cystic hyperplasia to almost 0% compared with 7% on oestrogen alone. Progestogen has also been shown to successfully treat women with proven endometrial cancers.

> The addition of progesterone to HRT regimes reduces the risk of endometrial carcinoma

With regard to the long-term use of sequential regimes, it appears that the risk of developing endometrial cancer increases, although to a lesser degree than if using unopposed oestrogen. Published studies are conflicting: some show a relative risk of up to 1.6 of developing endometrial cancer if using sequential HRT and others show no increase in risk. It may be that the risk is related to length of progesterone use, with a minimum of 12–14 days required to protect the endometrium.

It is too early to comment on the effects of continuous combined preparations on rates of endometrial cancer, but it seems likely that continuous administration of progesterone is the optimal method of protecting the endometrium in the long-term. The daily dose of progesterone produces an atrophic endometrium and lower rates of endometrial hyperplasia when compared to sequential preparations. Very low rates of hyperplasia are also seen for the levonorgestrel-secreting intrauterine system (LNG-IUS) which provides local progesterone-mediated endometrial suppression. The Women's Health Initiative (WHI) used a continuous combined preparation for an average of 5.2 years of follow-up. It is reassuring that the rates of endometrial cancer were slightly lower in the HRT group than in the placebo group.

> Continuous combined HRT preparations are probably the optimal way of protecting the endometrium in the long-term

Investigation of the endometrium

The incidence of endometrial cancer is very low prior to the age of 40 and rises steeply in the years approaching the menopause. Vaginal bleeding after the menopause is considered to be indicative of endometrial cancer until proven otherwise. However, most women who experience postmenopausal bleeding have no pathology or benign lesions.

> Vaginal bleeding after the menopause is considered to be indicative of endometrial cancer until proven otherwise

Unusual bleeding on HRT is one of the commonest reasons why women undergo investigation of the endometrium. The majority of these women are those who have unexpected bleeding on continuous combined preparations:

- If a woman experiences bleeding for the first 6 months of a continuous combined HRT course, this is likely to be a preparation-related effect on the endometrium. Such bleeding should be managed conservatively and changing preparations at an early stage is unlikely to be helpful.
- If the bleeding continues beyond 6 months, the chances of obtaining a bleed-free state are low and there is little point in continuing without further assessment. If

an underlying cause is excluded, then an alternative preparation can be useful. A lower dose of oestradiol, higher dose of progesterone or changing to tibolone should be considered.

- If a woman has been amenorrhoeic for several months and then experiences vaginal bleeding, this should be considered as postmenopausal bleeding and investigated accordingly.

It was believed that women on sequential HRT who experienced regular vaginal bleeding after the eleventh day of taking progesterone had a low risk of endometrial abnormality. However, as it is now known that the pattern of withdrawal bleeding does not correlate with endometrial hyperplasia, a regular bleed should not necessarily be interpreted as a reassuring sign.

Assessment of the endometrium is not routinely required prior to commencing HRT. However, women who are using sequential HRT for more than 5 years should be considered at a higher risk of developing endometrial cancer than those who have never used HRT or users of continuous combined therapy. If a woman opts to use sequential HRT in the long-term, then she should be considered for endometrial assessment.

> Women taking sequential HRT for more than 5 years should be considered at higher risk of developing endometrial cancer

HRT for women with endometrial cancer

Endometrial cancer is an oestrogen-sensitive malignancy and HRT is considered to be contraindicated once the diagnosis has been made. It may be that HRT can be considered in early tumours; however, there is even less evidence for use of HRT in endometrial cancer than there is with breast cancer (see below). Women with endometrial cancer require individual consideration of the risks and benefits in the context of a specialist clinic.

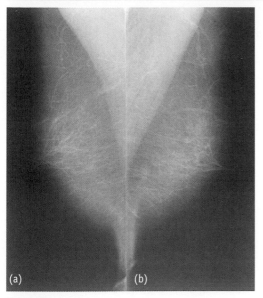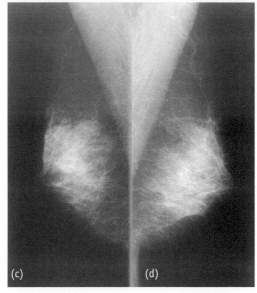

Figure 9.2
Changes in mammographic density after continuous combined postmenopausal HRT. Parts (a) and (b) show left and right breasts before HRT and parts (c) and (d) show left and right breasts after 4 months of therapy. (Images courtesy of Dr Carolyn Cordiner, West of Scotland Breast Screening Service.)

Breast cancer

As with the endometrium, the breast tissues proliferate in response to oestrogens (Figure 9.2). Unfortunately, there is no corresponding suppression for the breast tissue by progesterone as there is in the endometrium. Instead, progesterone also appears to have a stimulatory effect, increasing breast lobule development and epithelial cell differentiation.

Breast cancer is now the most commonly diagnosed malignancy in the UK and by age 74, one in nine women will have developed it. Unsurprisingly, it is a major concern for women in the developed world. The diagnosis of the condition has increased over recent years, probably due in part to increased levels of screening.

The issue of breast cancer and HRT remains emotive but careful explanation of the facts allows women to make informed choices. Observational data have shown that HRT confers a small, but significant, increased risk of developing breast cancer with long-term use. However, this increase in risk is often overestimated by women who may be considering taking HRT. It is helpful to compare the background level of breast cancer when considering the additional risk that HRT confers. This increased risk equates to an additional 2.3% for each year of use of HRT and this declines to almost normal levels 5 years after HRT is stopped (Table 9.1). Years of HRT use appear to equate to years of natural female hormones, ie a women who has an early menopause without HRT will have a lower risk of breast cancer than a women who has a later menopause.

There is some suggestion that the addition of progestogen may increase the risk of breast cancer to a greater extent than use of oestrogen alone; however, further studies are required. The WHI, a randomized trial of HRT for women with a uterus and ERT for women without a uterus, has recently stopped the HRT arm of the study due to increased rates of breast cancer (38/10,000 women years for HRT and 30/10,000 women years for placebo). The oestrogen-only arm of the trial has continued. Up to 10% of breast cancer cases in Western countries are related to genetic predisposition. As yet, there is no evidence that HRT increases these risks, however, women with a family history of breast cancer will require careful counselling with regard to HRT use.

These risks are generally thought to apply to years beyond the average age of menopause of 51. A woman with an early menopause may require many years of HRT before she reaches the age of 51 and she should consider this as replacement of natural hormone levels.

> Long-term HRT use confers a small, but significant, increased risk of breast cancer; this is often overestimated by women

There is no evidence of an increased mortality from breast cancer for HRT users and some studies have reported a lower mortality for breast cancer patients who use HRT. There is some evidence that breast cancers are diagnosed earlier in women on HRT. This is possibly because of increased vigilance among women and their doctors, but it may be that the tumours that develop under the influence of hormones are naturally less aggressive. Women with breast cancer who are prescribed HRT may also have less aggressive malignancies than those who are refused HRT.

HRT for women with breast cancer

Once a diagnosis of breast cancer has been made, the issue of HRT use becomes more controversial. The question of whether HRT is safe for use in women with breast cancer remains unanswered.

The traditional belief is that HRT use will increase the risk of recurrence of cancer. It is unlikely that female hormones directly initiate cancerous changes in cells. Both oestrogen and progesterone increase the activity of breast cells, thus potentially increasing the vulnerability of normal cells to mitotic effects

and potentially increasing the growth of existing tumours. Oestrogen-deprivation states, such as oophorectomy or the use of tamoxifen (an oestrogen antagonist), increase survival.

However, the evidence for an increased recurrence with HRT is scanty. Breast cancer was initially treated with stillboestrol. A randomized controlled trial of tamoxifen versus stillboestrol showed that tamoxifen was better tolerated, but rates of recurrence were similar in both groups. High levels of oestrogen during pregnancy do not appear to have a negative effect on the survival of women who also have breast cancer, which is reassuring when considering the use of HRT.

The treatment modalities chemotherapy and radiotherapy can predispose women to a premature menopause. The avoidance of HRT for women with breast cancer may put them at higher risk of developing diseases associated with the menopause, in particular osteoporosis. Although tamoxifen acts as an oestrogen antagonist in the breast it also has an agonist effect in other tissues. There is evidence that tamoxifen protects against osteoporosis, but this oestrogenic effect can also lead to hyperplastic changes within the endometrium and women on tamoxifen are at greater risk of developing endometrial cancer.

Small case-control studies have shown no evidence of a detrimental effect in women with breast cancer who use HRT. The numbers are small and it may be that women with more favourable prognoses are more likely to receive HRT. Randomized controlled trials of use of HRT in women with breast cancer are in progress.

Although there is little definite evidence of harm, it is entirely appropriate that use of oestrogen to treat menopausal symptoms in women with breast cancer is approached with a degree of caution. Several factors need to be considered when making a decision about HRT, ideally in consultation with the breast surgeon involved (Table 9.2). It would also be

Table 9.2
Factors to consider in prescribing HRT to women with breast cancer

- Age
- Aggressiveness of the tumour
- Time since diagnosis
- Oestrogen receptor status
- Severity of vasomotor symptoms
- Quality of life
- Risk factors for osteoporosis
- Risk factors for cardiovascular disease

reasonable to try alternatives such as progestogens, clonidine or venlafaxine before embarking on the use of oestrogen-based HRT.

Ovarian cancer

HRT users may have a higher risk of ovarian cancer. Not all studies have shown this association and it may be that other factors are confounding. A North American study questioned a large cohort of women about oestrogen use in 1982. Ovarian cancer deaths were then recorded over the next 14 years of follow up. It found a relative risk of 1.51 of dying of ovarian cancer for oestrogen users at baseline. Ongoing use of oestrogen for all participants was not assessed and the relationship between HRT and ovarian cancer was not examined.

Malignant melanoma

The relationship between melanoma and HRT is conflicting. There is no evidence that HRT has a significant relationship with the development of the disease. However, the fact that oestrogen receptors are found on melanoma cells does cause concern. If possible, HRT is best avoided within the first 2 years when most recurrences occur.

The association between HRT and malignancy has been evolving for many years. With continued research we might be able to reduce the risks; however, the decision to use or prescribe HRT must be based on current available evidence. Increasingly, the role of the medical practitioner is to interpret and relate evidence to the patient as an individual.

Further reading

Beral V, Bull D, Doll R et al. The Collaborative Group on Hormonal Factors in Breast Cancer. Breast cancer and hormone replacement therapy: collaborative reanalysis of data from 51 epidemiological studies of 527505 women with breast cancer and 108411 women without breast cancer. Lancet 1997; **350**: 1047–59.

Beresford SA, Weiss NS, Voigt LF, McKnight B. Risk of endometrial cancer in relation to use of oestrogen combined with cyclic progestagen therapy in postmenopausal women. Lancet 1997; **349**: 458–61.

Bergman L, Bellen MLR, Gallee MPW et al. Risk and prognosis of endometrial cancer after tamoxifen for breast cancer. Lancet 2000; **356**: 881–7.

Bergvist L, Adami H-G, Persson I et al. Prognosis after breast cancer diagnosis in women exposed to estrogen-progestogen replacement therapy. Am J Epidemiol 1989; **130**: 221–8.

Col NF, Hirota LK, Orr RK et al. Hormone replacement therapy after breast cancer: a systematic review and quantitative assessment of risk. J Clin Oncol 2001; **19**: 2357–63.

Colditz GA, Egan KM. Hormone replacement therapy and the risk of breast cancer: results from epidemiologic studies. Am J Obstet Gynecol 1993; **168**: 1473–80.

Gapstur SM, Morrow M, Sellers TA. Hormone replacement therapy and the risk of breast cancer with a favourable histology: results of the Iowa women's health study. JAMA 1999; **281**: 2091–7.

Goodwin PJ, Ennis M, Pritchard KI et al. Risk of menopause during the first year after breast cancer diagnosis. J Clin Oncol 1999; **17**: 2365–70.

Grady D, Gebretsadik T, Kerlikowske K et al. Hormone replacement therapy and endometrial cancer risk: a meta-analysis. Obstet Gynecol 1995; **85**: 304–13.

Herrinton LJ, Weiss NS. Postmenopausal unopposed estrogens. Characteristics of use in relation to the risk of endometrial carcinoma. Ann Epidemiol 1993; **3**: 308–18.

McPherson K, Steel CM, Dixon JM. Breast cancer, epidemiology, risk factors and genetics. Br Med J 2000; **321**: 624–8.

Rodriguez C, Patel AV, Calle EE et al. Estrogen replacement therapy and ovarian cancer mortality in a large prospective study of US women. JAMA 2001; **285**: 1460–5.

Shapiro JA, Weiss NS, Beresford SA, Voigt LF. Menopausal hormone use and endometrial cancer, by tumour grade and invasion. Epidemiology 1998; **9**: 99–101.

Sturdee DW, Ulrich LG, Barlow DH et al. The endometrial response to sequential and continuous combined oestrogen-progestogen replacement therapy. Br J Obstet Gynaecol 2000; **107**(11): 1392–400.

Sturdee DW, Barlow DH, Ulrich LG. Is the timing of withdrawal bleeding a guide to endometrial safety during sequential oestrogen-progestagen replacement therapy? UK Continuous Combined HRT Study Investigators. *Lancet* 1994; **344**: 979–82.

Weiderpass E, Adami HO, Baron JA *et al.* Risk of endometrial cancer following estrogen replacement with and without progestins. *J Natl Cancer Inst* 1999; **91**: 1131–7.

Wollter-Svensson LO, Stadberg E Andersson K *et al.* Intrauterine administration of levonorgestrel 5 and 10 microg/24 hours in perimenopausal hormone replacement therapy. A randomised clinical trial during one year. *Acta Obstet Gynecol Scand* 1997; **776**: 449–54.

Writing group for the Women's Health Initiative. Risks and benefits of estrogen plus progestin in healthy postmenopausal women. *JAMA* 2002; **288**: 321–33.

Index

Page numbers in *italics* refer to information that is shown only in a table or diagram.

absorptiometry, for osteoporosis assessment 40
acne, with progestogens 32
administration of HRT
  comparison of routes *25*
  nasal administration 26–7
  oral oestrogens 24–5
  progestogens 27
  subcutaneous implants 26
  transdermal administration *see* transdermal HRT
    administration
  vaginal administration *see* vaginal HRT administration
adverse effects of HRT *see* side-effects of HRT
age at menopause, factors influencing 3
age, menstrual cycle changes with 5–6
alendronate, for osteoporosis 45–7
alpha-blockers, for vasomotor symptoms 11
alternative therapies 27–8
Alzheimer's disease, and HRT 33
androgens, and sexual function 15
anovulatory cycles 6–7
antidepressants, for vasomotor symptoms 11
anxiety, as symptom of menopause 13–14
arterial disease
  blood pressure and HRT 52
  HRT in high CHD risk women 53
  HRT recommendations 52–3
  protective effects of HRT 49
  risk factors 49–52
assisted conception, and premature ovarian failure 19
autoimmune disorders, and premature ovarian failure
  17

biochemical markers, for osteoporosis assessment 40
bisphosphonates, for osteoporosis treatment
  45–7
bloating, with progestogens 32
blood pressure, HRT effects on 34, 52
bone mass, and osteoporosis risk 38–9
bone mineral density (BMD), osteoporosis assessment
  40–2
bone remodelling 37–8
breast cancer, and HRT 62–5
breast tenderness, with progestogens 32

C-reactive protein, HRT effects on
  and cardiovascular disease risk *51*, 52
  oral oestrogens 24–5

  and VTE risk 56
calcitonin
  and bone remodelling 38
  for osteoporosis 47
calcium, for osteoporosis 43
cancer
  breast cancer 62–5
  and compliance with HRT 31
  endometrial cancer 61–2
  malignant melanoma 65
  ovarian cancer 65
cardiovascular disease
  blood pressure and HRT 52
  HRT in high CHD risk women 53
  HRT recommendations 52–3
  and premature ovarian failure 18–19
  protective effects of HRT 49
  risk factors 49–52
cerebrovascular disease, and HRT 34–5
chemotherapy, and premature ovarian failure *17*, 19
cholesterol levels, HRT effects on
  and cardiovascular disease risk 50–1
  oral oestrogens 24–5
cigarette smoking
  and age at menopause 3
  and premature ovarian failure *17*
clonidine, for vasomotor symptoms 11
clotting factors, HRT effects on 51–2
coagulation, HRT effects on
  and cardiovascular disease risk 51–2
  oral oestrogens 24–5
  and VTE risk 56
cognitive symptoms 14
combined oral contraceptive pill, for hormone
  replacement 19–20
compliance with HRT 30–1
computed tomography, for osteoporosis assessment
  40
concentration, loss of, as symptom of menopause 14
conjugated equine oestrogens (Premarin) 24
  and cardiovascular disease risk 49–50
  HERS study 50–1
continuous combined HRT therapy 23
  endometrial cancer risk with 61–2
  vaginal bleeding with 31
contraception, in perimenopause 19
contraindications to HRT use 32–3

coronary heart disease (CHD)
    protective effects of HRT 49
    risk factors 49–52
cultural differences, in symptoms of menopause 10

definitions
    age at menopause 3
    menopause 2–3
    perimenopause 3
    premature menopause 3–4
dementia, and HRT 33
densitometry techniques, for osteoporosis assessment
    40
depression, as symptom of menopause 13–14
desogestrel 27
DEXA (dual-energy X-ray absorptiometry), for
    osteoporosis assessment 40, 41
diabetes, and HRT 37
dietary supplements 28
1,25-dihydroxyvitamin D, and bone remodelling 38
dydrogesterone 27

education, and HRT uptake 30
embryo cryoperservation, and premature ovarian failure
    19
endometrial cancer
    and HRT 61–2
    HRT use in women with 62
    investigations 62
endometrial hyperplasia, and HRT 61
endometriosis, and HRT 33–4
epilepsy, and HRT 34
equine oestrogens (Premarin) see conjugated equine
    oestrogens (Premarin)
Estring, vaginal oestradiol administration 26
ethinyl oestradiol 24
etidronate, for osteoporosis treatment 45–7

fertility, and premature ovarian failure 19
fibrinolysis, HRT effects on
    and cardiovascular disease risk 51–2
    oral oestrogens 24–5
    and VTE risk 56
first-pass metabolism
    of oral oestrogens 24–5
    and subcutaneous implants 26
    and transdermal oestrogens 25–6
fluid retention, with progestogens 32
fluoride, and bone remodelling 38
follicle-stimulating hormone (FSH)
    age-related changes 5–6
    and menopause diagnosis 7
    and ovarian physiology 4–5
    perimenopausal changes 7
    and premature ovarian failure diagnosis 17–18
follicles, premature depletion of see premature ovarian
    failure (POF)
fracture risk, and osteoporosis see osteoporosis

gel preparations
    of oestrogens 25–6
    see also transdermal HRT administration
genetic disorders, and premature ovarian failure 17
genital tract symptoms 12–13
glucocorticoids, and bone remodelling 38
gonadal cryopreservation, and premature ovarian failure
    19
gonadotrophins see follicle-stimulating hormone (FSH);
    luteinizing hormone (LH)
greasy skin, with progestogens 32
Greene's Menopause Scale 21, 22
growth hormone, and bone remodelling 38

HDL-cholesterol, HRT effects on
    and cardiovascular disease risk 50–1
    oral oestrogens 24–5
headache
    with progestogens 32
    as symptom of menopause 12
healthy user bias
    and HRT benefits 30
    HRT effects on coronary heart disease 47
herbal remedies 28
HERS study (Heart and Estrogen/Progestin Replacement
    Study)
    and cardiovascular disease risk 49–50, 50–1
    and VTE risk 55
history 1–2
hormone replacement therapy (HRT) see HRT
hot flushes 10–11
HRT
    alternatives to 27–8
    and blood pressure 34, 52
    and breast cancer 62–5
    and cardiovascular disease 49–53
    for cognitive symptoms 14
    compliance 30–1
    contraindications 32–3
    and dementia 33
    and diabetes 37
    and endometrial cancer 61–2
    and endometriosis 33–4
    and epilepsy 34
    follow-up consultation 23
    and headache management 12
    history 2
    and hypertension 34
    investigations 21
    and malignant melanoma 65
    and menopausal symptoms 21
    menopause consultation 21–3
    and migraine 34
    oestrogen administration routes 24–7
    oestrogen types 24
    for osteoporosis treatment 43–5
    and otosclerosis 34
    and ovarian cancer 65

for premature ovarian failure 19–20
preparations 23–4
prescribing 21–2
progestogens 27
risk:benefit assessment 21
side-effects *see* side-effects of HRT
and stroke 34–5
and systemic lupus erythematosus 33
uptake of 29, 30
for urogenital symptoms 12–13
vaginal bleeding with 23–4
for vasomotor symptoms 11
and venous thromboembolism 55–8
hydroxyprogesterone 27
hypertension, and HRT 34
hysterectomy
and age at menopause 4
and premature ovarian failure *17*

in-vitro fertilization (IVF), and premature ovarian failure 19
infertility, and premature ovarian failure 19
inflammation, HRT effects on
and cardiovascular disease risk *51*, 52
and VTE risk 56
inhibin, age-related changes 6
insomnia 11
isoflavones 28

LDL-cholesterol, HRT effects on
and cardiovascular disease risk 50–1
oral oestrogens 24–5
levonorgestrel, oral administration 27
levonorgestrel-secreting intrauterine system (LNG-IUS) 27
endometrial cancer risk with 62
and vaginal bleeding 31–2
libido, loss of, as symptom of menopause 14–15
life expectancy, and menopause 1
lipid levels, HRT effects on
and cardiovascular disease risk 50–1
oral oestrogens 24–5
long cycle HRT therapy 23
luteinizing hormone (LH)
and menopause diagnosis 7
and ovarian physiology 4–5
perimenopausal changes 7

malignant melanoma, and HRT 65
medroxyprogesterone
and cardiovascular disease risk 49–50
HERS study 50–1
in high CHD risk women 53
lipid changes with 51
oral administration 27
memory impairment, as symptom of menopause 14
menopausal symptoms *see* symptoms
menopausal transition *see* perimenopause
menopause
age at 3

definition 2–3
historical perspective 1–2
physiology 6–7
menopause consultation 21–3
Menoring, vaginal oestradiol administration 26
menstrual cycle
perimenopausal changes 6–7
physiology 5–6
mestranol 24
metabolic effects of HRT
and cardiovascular disease risk 50–2
oral oestrogens 24–5
migraine 12
and HRT 34
mood changes, as symptom of menopause 13–14

nasal oestrogen administration *25*, 26–7
night sweats 11
norethisterone
in high CHD risk women 53
lipid changes with 51
oral administration 27
norgestimate 27
norgestrel 27
Nurses study, HRT effects on coronary heart disease 49

oestradiol
in high CHD risk women 53
in HRT preparations 24
lipid changes with 50
metabolic effects *51*
nasal administration 26–7
perimenopausal changes 7
and premature ovarian failure diagnosis 17–18
and stroke 34–5
subcutaneous implants 26
transdermal preparations 25–6
oestriol, in HRT preparations 24
oestrogen-only HRT 23
endometrial cancer risk with 61
oestrogens
and bone remodelling 38
and breast cancer risk 62–5
and dementia 33
for depression 14
endometrial cancer risk with 61
in high CHD risk women 53
in HRT preparations 24
for mood changes 13–14
nasal administration 26–7
oral administration 24–5
for osteoporosis treatment 43–5
perimenopausal changes 7
and stroke 34–5
subcutaneous implants 26
transdermal administration 25–6
vaginal administration 26
and vasomotor symptoms 11

oestrone
  in HRT preparations 24
  perimenopausal changes 7
oestropipate, in HRT preparations *24*
oocyte donation, and premature ovarian failure 19
oophorectomy, and premature ovarian failure *17*
oral contraceptives, for hormone replacement 19–20
oral HRT administration
  and cardiovascular disease 49–52
  oestrogens 24–5
  progestogens 27
osteopenia 40, *41*
osteoporosis
  diagnosis 39–40
  and fracture incidence 37
  pathogenesis 37–8
  and premature ovarian failure 18
  risk factors 38–9
  screening and prevention 40–2
  treatment 42–7
ovarian cancer, and HRT 65
ovarian physiology 4–5

parathyroid hormone, and bone remodelling 38
patch preparations
  of oestrogens 25–6
  see also transdermal HRT administration
peak bone mass, and osteoporosis risk 38–9
perimenopause
  definition 3
  and fertility 19
physiology
  menopause 6–7
  menstruation 5–6
  ovarian functions 4–5
phytoestrogens 28
Premarin (conjugated equine oestrogens) 24
  and cardiovascular disease risk 49–50
  HERS study 50–1
premature menopause 3–4
premature ovarian failure (POF)
  and cardiovascular disease 18–19
  causes 17
  diagnosis 17–18
  and fertility 19
  hormone replacement therapy 19–20
  and osteoporosis 18
  psychological effects 18
progesterone, administration routes 27
progestogens
  administration routes 27
  and breast cancer 62–5
  and endometrial cancer 61–2
  and headache 12
  in high CHD risk women 53
  lipid changes with 51
  for osteoporosis treatment 45
  side-effects of 32–3

for vasomotor symptoms 11
psychological effects, of premature ovarian failure 18

racial differences, in symptoms of menopause 10
radiotherapy, and premature ovarian failure *17*, 19
raloxifene 27, 45
resistant ovary syndrome *see* premature ovarian failure
  (POF)
risedronate, for osteoporosis 45–7
risk:benefit assessment
  and compliance with HRT 30–1
  and HRT uptake 30

selective oestrogen receptor modulators (SERMs) 27, 45
sequential HRT therapy 23
  endometrial cancer risk with 61
  progestogenic side-effects 32
sexual function problems, as symptom of menopause
  14–15
side-effects of HRT
  and compliance 30–1
  and HRT uptake 29
  oral oestrogens 24–5
  progestogenic effects 27, 32–3
  vaginal bleeding 31–2
  weight gain 32
skin greasiness, with progestogens 32
sleep disturbance 11
smoking
  and age at menopause 3
  and premature ovarian failure *17*
socioeconomic factors
  and HRT uptake 30
  and symptoms of menopause 9
soy isoflavones 28
stroke, and HRT 34–5
subcutaneous oestrogen implants *25*, 26
surgical menopause 4
symptoms 9
  anxiety and depression 13–14
  concentration and memory impairment 14
  headache 12
  loss of libido 14–15
  and menopause consultation 21, 22
  racial and cultural differences 10
  socioeconomic influences 9
  urinary symptoms 12–13
  vaginal atrophy 12–13
  vasomotor symptoms 10–11
synthetic oestrogens 24
systemic lupus erythematosus (SLE), and HRT 33

tachyphylaxis, with oestradiol implants 26
tamoxifen 27, 45
testosterone
  and sexual function 15
  subcutaneous implants 26
thrombophilia, and VTE risk 56